NEW DIRECTIONS FOR N

H. Richard Lamb, *University of Southern California*
EDITOR-IN-CHIEF

Dual Diagnosis of Major Mental Illness and Substance Disorder

Kenneth Minkoff
Choate Health Systems
Harvard Medical School

Robert E. Drake
Dartmouth Medical School

EDITORS

Number 50, Summer 1991

JOSSEY-BASS INC., PUBLISHERS, San Francisco

MAXWELL MACMILLAN INTERNATIONAL PUBLISHING GROUP
New York • Oxford • Singapore • Sydney • Toronto

DUAL DIAGNOSIS OF MAJOR MENTAL ILLNES AND SUBSTANCE DISORDER
Kenneth Minkoff, Robert E. Drake (eds.)
New Directions for Mental Health Services, no. 50
H. Richard Lamb, Editor-in-Chief

Microfilm copies of issues and articles are available in 16mm and 35mm,
as well as microfiche in 105mm, through University Microfilms Inc., 300
North Zeeb Road, Ann Arbor, Michigan 48106.

LC 87-646993   ISSN 0193-9416   ISBN 1-55542-794-4

NEW DIRECTIONS FOR MENTAL HEALTH SERVICES is part of The Jossey-
Bass Social and Behavioral Sciences Series and is published quarterly by
Jossey-Bass Inc., Publishers, 350 Sansome Street, San Francisco, Califor-
nia 94104-1310 (publication number USPS 493-910). Second-class post-
age paid at San Francisco, California, and at additional mailing offices.
POSTMASTER: Send address changes to New Directions for Mental Health
Services, Jossey-Bass Inc., Publishers, 350 Sansome Street, San Francisco,
California 94104-1310.

EDITORIAL CORRESPONDENCE should be sent to the Editor-in-Chief,
H. Richard Lamb, Department of Psychiatry and the Behavioral Sciences,
U.S.C. School of Medicine, 1934 Hospital Place, Los Angeles, California
90033.

Cover photograph by Wernher Krutein/PHOTOVAULT © 1990.

The paper used in this journal is acid-free and meets the strictest
guidelines in the United States for recycled paper (50 percent
recycled waste, including 10 percent post-consumer waste).
Manufactured in the United States of America.

CONTENTS

EDITORS' NOTES

The widespread prevalence of substance disorders (both substance abuse and dependence) in patients suffering from serious mental illnesses (schizophrenia, major affective disorders, and other psychoses) has been increasingly well documented in the past decade. In many settings, the presence of such "dual diagnoses" in the treatment population is so common that it must be considered to be an expectation, rather than an exception.

The problems associated with providing effective treatment for dual diagnosis patients involve more than their sheer numbers, however. Dual diagnosis patients are frequently "system misfits" who have difficulty both in accessing services and in accepting services. Clinicians, program managers, and system planners find them to be difficult patients who are resistant and nonresponsive to traditional interventions. Moreover, dual diagnosis patients have been repeatedly demonstrated to have poorer outcomes in almost every sphere; they have more relapses and rehospitalizations, poorer treatment compliance, more acting out behavior, and increased risk of homelessness.

Although there has been fairly extensive research describing and documenting the clinical characteristics of the dual diagnosis population, little controlled research is available so far to guide clinical treatment or program development. Nonetheless, the pressing need for dual diagnosis services is becoming more and more urgent.

In the past few years there have been significant advances in both the conceptualization and the development of innovative program models providing integrated assessment and concomitant treatment for dually disordered patients. The purpose of this volume is to provide the reader with information about the most current ideas and clinical interventions available. Although many of the models presented have been successful only in clinical trials, and efficacy is not yet confirmed by controlled research, the principles used in the development of those models will hopefully have value in assisting clinicians, managers, and planners who have an immediate need to provide services to this population.

The volume begins with an overview of the dual diagnosis problem, and then proceeds with a discussion of the general principles involved in designing a continuous, comprehensive, and integrated care system for dual diagnosis patients. Common characteristics of successful hybrid programs are described next, followed by an up-to-date analysis of the progress and technology of assessment. The final four chapters are descriptions of specific innovative program models, each unique and potentially replicable: a comprehensive continuum of services developed in New Hampshire, with statewide intensive case management; a replicable modular program for step-by-step engagement of dual diagnosis patients in substance treatment that can be adapted to any program setting; a creative dual diagnosis residential treatment program in New York City, developed in a traditional *addiction* therapeutic community; and a discussion of alternative models for providing effective dual diagnosis services to the homeless mentally ill.

Kenneth Minkoff
Robert E. Drake
Editors

Kenneth Minkoff, M.D., is chief of psychiatric services at Choate Health Systems in Woburn, Mass., and medical director of the Caulfield Center, an integrated psychiatry and addiction hospital. He is on the clinical faculty of the Cambridge Hospital Department of Psychiatry of the Harvard Medical School.

Robert E. Drake, M.D., Ph.D., is associate professor of psychiatry at Dartmouth Medical School and director of the New Hampshire–Dartmouth Psychiatric Research Center.

Dual diagnosis of severe mental illness and substance disorder is a frequent and difficult challenge to the mental health and substance abuse systems. This chapter reviews the dual diagnosis problem and introduces the chapters that follow.

Dual Diagnosis of Major Mental Illness and Substance Disorder: An Overview

Robert E. Drake, Peggy McLaughlin,
Bert Pepper, Kenneth Minkoff

The phenomenon of co-occurring major mental illness and substance disorder is now widely recognized. The Epidemiologic Catchment Area (ECA) study (Regier and others, 1984) confirmed the extensive comorbidity of substance disorders with a wide range of psychiatric disorders, including the most severe disorders, in the community. One-month odds ratios in three sites showed that people with schizophrenia, for example, have a 10.1 times greater rate of alcohol use disorders and a 7.6 times greater rate of other drug use disorders than nonschizophrenic people (Boyd and others, 1984). A more recent analysis of the ECA data (Regier and others, 1990) supported the increased risk of substance abuse or dependence among those with severe mental illnesses. For example, 47 percent of individuals with a lifetime diagnosis of schizophrenia or schizophreniform disorder had met criteria for some form of substance abuse or dependence.

The ECA study also confirmed Berkson's bias (Berkson, 1946)—that individuals with comorbidity are more likely to be found in clinical samples. The rates of diagnosed comorbidity in clinical settings continue to rise as clinicians become more aware of the high prevalence and more skilled at identifying multiple disorders (Lehmann, Myers, and Corty, 1989). Over a third of patients in general psychiatric settings and half or more of those in settings that provide more intensive treatment, such as psychiatric emergency rooms or inpatient psychiatric programs, have problems substantially affected by substance abuse or dependence (Galanter, Castaneda, and Ferman, 1988).

Terminology

Despite several attempts to designate a simple label for the phenomenon of co-occurring severe psychiatric disorder and substance disorder (for example, chemical abusing mentally ill, comorbidity, dual diagnosis, dual disorder, mentally ill chemical abuser, mentally ill substance abuser, psychiatrically impaired substance abuser), no consensus has emerged around a single rubric. Perhaps the names proliferate because all are nonspecific. We believe that authors should at this time continue to specify in detail the population they are discussing. The chapters in this volume refer specifically to people with dual diagnoses of major mental illness (that is, severe and persistent psychiatric disorders that cause prolonged disability and require long-term care) and substance disorder (that is, abuse of or dependence on alcohol or other drugs).

Why Are Dual Diagnoses So Common?

To some extent, the increase in multiple diagnoses of alcohol, drug, and mental disorders in clinical settings is due to enhanced awareness. However, at least two factors—deinstitutionalization and changing patterns of drug use in the culture—have contributed to a real increase in the prevalence among treated populations.

First, an entire generation of young adults with major mental illness in the United States has grown up and become ill in the era of deinstitutionalization. Like previous cohorts of chronically mentally ill people, these young adults have few skills, many deficits, diverse symptoms, and extensive needs for psychiatric care and supportive services (Bachrach, 1982; Caton, 1981; Pepper, Kirshner, and Ryglewicz, 1981). Unlike previous cohorts, however, they receive most of their long-term treatment in the community rather than in hospitals (Minkoff, 1987) and so have ready access to alcohol and other drugs (Lamb, 1982; Pepper, Kirshner, and Ryglewicz, 1981; Robbins and others, 1978; Schwartz and Goldfinger, 1981).

Second, during the same years that the deinstitutionalization ideology has been implemented, social acceptance of and experimentation with illegal drugs has increased dramatically in the United States. In the early 1960s only 2 percent or less of the population had experimented with illegal drugs, but by 1982 almost one-third of the population over twelve had used these drugs (American Psychiatric Association, 1987), and by 1985 almost half of young adults had tried various substances of abuse other than alcohol (National Institute on Drug Abuse, 1987). Many young people abuse drugs for several years prior to the development of their psychiatric disorders (Barbee and others, 1989; Breakey, Goodell, Lorenz, and McHugh, 1974; Caton, Gralnick, Bender, and Simon, 1989) and are first treated in addiction centers. Furthermore, vulnerable young people have been exposed to new types of drugs (such as LSD in the 1960s, PCP in the 1970s, and potent forms of cocaine in the 1980s) that distort symptoms, obscure diagnosis, and adversely affect the course and treatment of major mental illness (Dixon and others, 1990).

Reasons for Use

People with major mental illnesses may begin to use alcohol and other drugs for the same reasons as others in society. Several additional factors have been hypothesized to contribute to the high rate of substance abuse and dependence in this population: downward social drift into living settings in poor urban areas in which drug use and purveyance are common (Lieberman and Bowers, 1990), misguided attempts to alleviate, or self-medicate, the symptoms of mental illness or the side effects of psychotropic medications (Schneier and Siris, 1987), attempts to develop an identity that is more acceptable than that of mental patient (Lamb, 1982), and attempts to facilitate social interactions (Bergman and Harris, 1985).

These hypotheses do not explain the heavy use of alcohol and other drugs prior to the onset of psychiatric symptoms that characterizes many people with chronic illnesses (Barbee and others, 1989; Breakey, Goodell, Lorenz, and McHugh, 1974; Caton, Gralnick, Bender, and Simon, 1989). For them, drugs may precipitate or induce psychiatric disorder (Bowers and Swigar, 1983; Breakey, Goodell, Lorenz, and McHugh, 1974; McLellan, Woody, and O'Brien, 1979). Painful internal states or interpersonal problems that exist prior to the onset of overt mental illness may be significant risk factors. Consistent with this view, schizophrenic patients typically report that alcohol and other drugs of abuse reduce dysphoria, anxiety, and social problems rather than psychotic symptoms (Dixon and others, 1990; Noordsy and others, in press).

We lack prospective research data regarding the onset and development of substance disorder and severe mental illness. Popular explanations that involve self-medication may well represent post hoc rationalizations on the part of dually diagnosed patients and their caregivers. In any case, early experimentation and the immediate effects of alcohol and other drugs should be differentiated from the factors that sustain problematic use. Biological reinforcement mechanisms, related learning phenomena, and the lack of significant social and material resources may account for sustained abuse and dependence independently of the reasons for initial use. We actually know little about etiology, and the recent psychiatric literature reflects the view that comorbid substance disorders should be considered independent and autonomous problems rather than secondary disorders (Lehmann, Myers, and Corty, 1989; Minkoff, 1989; Osher and Kofoed, 1989).

Course and Outcome

Longitudinal data regarding the course and outcome of comorbid severe mental illness and substance disorder are meager (Turner and Tsuang, 1990). Cross-sectional studies indicate that substance abuse among people with major mental illness is associated with more severe psychiatric symptoms (Barbee and others, 1989; Carey, Carey, and Meisler, in press; Osher and others, 1991); disruptive behaviors (Alterman, Erdlin, McLellan, and Mann, 1980; McCarrick, Manderscheid, and Bertolucci, 1985; Safer, 1987), including verbal hostility (Alterman, Erdlin, McLellan, and Mann, 1980; Drake and Wallach, 1989), aggression (Yesavage and Zarcone, 1983), and criminal behavior (Safer, 1987; Schutt and Garrett, 1988); and suicidal behavior (Drake, Osher, and Wallach, 1989; Kesselman, Solomon, Beaudett, and Thornton, 1982). The dually diagnosed also have more difficulty managing the practical aspects of their lives (Alterman, Erdlin, McLellan, and Mann, 1980; Drake, Osher, and Wallach, 1989; Safer, 1987). They are particularly prone to problems with housing instability and homelessness (Benda and Dattalo, 1988; Drake and Wallach, 1989; Drake and others, in press; Lamb, 1984). They tend to be treatment noncompliant (Alterman, Erdlin, McLellan, and Mann, 1980; Drake and Wallach, 1989; Richardson, Craig, and Haugland, 1985) or not in treatment at all. A large proportion of the homeless mentally ill have had no recent contacts with the mental health system whatsoever, even if they are extremely disabled (Bassuk, Rubin, and Lauriat, 1984; Kroll and others, 1986; Roth and Bean, 1986). Similarly, the ECA study in three sites found that about half of those with a current diagnosis of schizophrenia or schizophreniform disorder had had no contact with mental health caregivers in the previous six months (Regier and Burke, 1987). The dually diagnosed are also prone to institutionalization in hospitals and jails (Drake and Wallach, 1989; Lamb and Grant, 1982; Osher and others, 1991; Safer, 1987).

Whether disrupting the mental health system or avoiding it, these individuals are clearly different from the passive, compliant persons with major mental illness who were deinstitutionalized in the 1950s and 1960s (Minkoff, 1987). They do not fit readily into the existing mental health or substance abuse treatment systems (Group for the Advancement of Psychiatry, 1987; Ridgely, Osher, and Talbott, 1987; Schwartz and Goldfinger, 1981; Solomon, 1986–87).

Federal Response

Clinicians, treatment programs, and treatment systems began to respond to the changing realities of the culture and the patients in the early 1980s. The Alcohol, Drug Abuse, and Mental Health Administration (ADAMHA) sponsored a conference in 1982 that identified coexisting major mental illness and substance disorder as a major problem. In 1985 ADAMHA commissioned a series of reports by the University of Maryland on the problems of young adults with chronic mental illness and substance abuse problems. Ridgely, Talbott, Goldman, and Osher reviewed the literature and studied programs in different areas of the country in order to identify needs related to treatment, training, and research (Ridgely, Goldman, and Talbott, 1986; Ridgely, Osher, and Talbott, 1987). These reports addressed numerous administrative barriers, resistances, and gaps within the substance abuse and mental health service systems.

The reviews by Ridgely and colleagues emphasized that most mental health and substance abuse treatment systems were not addressing the dual diagnosis problem effectively. Individuals with co-occurring substance disorder and severe psychiatric disorder had worse outcomes than individuals with either disorder alone, in part because of the failure of the treatment systems to respond to their needs appropriately. Standard care involved extrusion from both systems (because of the other disorder), sequential treatment (that is, stabilized in one system and then referred to the other), or treatment in parallel systems with little coordination. Caregivers were typically trained in one discipline—mental health or chemical dependency—without much knowledge or experience with the other perspective.

Development of Integrated Treatment Models

In the past few years, clinicians and others have advocated for mental health and substance abuse treatments that are concurrent and integrated (Drake, Teague, and Warren, 1990; Lehmann, Myers, and Corty, 1989; Minkoff, 1989; Osher and Kofoed, 1989; Ridgely, Osher, and Talbott, 1987). Initial attempts at integration have been demonstrably effective in open clinical trials (Hellerstein and Meehan, 1987; Kofoed, Kania, Walsh, and Atkinson, 1986). As Kline and colleagues discuss in this volume, integration can occur through hybrid programs or through careful linkage by case managers. Integration needs to occur at the treatment level, the program level, and the system level.

In the context of a growing awareness that integrated treatment might be more effective, the NIMH Community Support Program funded thirteen demonstration programs in 1987 for young adults with mental health and substance abuse problems (Teague, Schwab, and Drake, 1990). These thirteen programs examined a rich variety of approaches to linking the two treatment systems to enhance services for the dually diagnosed. Some programs concentrated on system linkage, some on integrating one set of services within the other system's program, and still others on creating a separate hybrid program outside of the existing mental health and substance abuse programs. The demonstration programs endeavored to learn more about the treatment needs of the dually diagnosed, to discover ways of breaking down service system barriers, to examine the advantages and disadvantages of different ways of linking the systems, and to explore training and human resource development issues more generally.

Since 1987 the three component institutes of ADAMHA—NIMH, NIAAA, and NIDA—have funded numerous clinical research demonstrations and research projects focused on dual diagnosis of major mental illness and substance disorder. These emphasize different subgroups, such as the homeless, adolescents, minorities, and women. They also emphasize a variety of inpatient and outpatient treatment approaches. Within the next five years, as results continue to accumulate from these studies, our understanding of those with dual disorders and of effective treatments will advance considerably.

Current State of the Art

While we await the results of controlled investigations, clinical experience in the evaluation and treatment of dually diagnosed patients is rapidly growing, and administrative guidelines for linking systems and effecting philosophical and system changes are steadily emerging. This volume summarizes the current state of knowledge for clinicians and program developers. Clinicians and researchers who have been active in the dual diagnosis field for several years discuss assessment (Kofoed), conceptualization of treatment systems (Minkoff), and model programs (Ridgely), and also provide examples of current programs in the mental health system (Drake and colleagues; Kline and colleagues; Sciacca) and in the chemical dependency system (Pepper and McLaughlin).

The chapters that follow describe the most current clinical approaches to dual diagnosis patients, and, in doing so, specifically address many of the dilemmas and controversies in the field:

- When should treatment be integrated rather than concurrent and parallel?
- How can the twelve-step program be combined with mental health treatment?
- How should medications be used in chemical dependency treatment?
- When and for whom should treatment focus on abstinence rather than controlled drinking?
- Should one disorder be considered primary and the other secondary?
- How can conflicting treatment philosophies in the mental health and substance abuse systems be resolved?
- When should we develop new programs, and when should we modify existing ones?

These questions obviously need careful research. Nevertheless, current concepts and models, derived from successful programs, provide pragmatic solutions for the pressing need to provide services.

References

Alterman, A. I., Erdlin, F. R., McLellan, A. T., and Mann, S. C. "Problem Drinking in Hospitalized Schizophrenic Patients." *Addictive Behaviors*, 1980, *5*, 273–276.

American Psychiatric Association, Committee on Drug Abuse. "Position Statement on Psychoactive Substance Use and Dependence: Update on Marijuana and Cocaine." *American Journal of Psychiatry*, 1987, *144*, 698–701.

Bachrach, L. L. "Young Adult Chronic Patients: An Analytical Review of the Literature." *Hospital and Community Psychiatry*, 1982, *33*, 189–197.

Barbee, J. G., Clark, P. D., Crapanzano, M. S., Heintz, G. C., and Kehoe, C. E. "Alcohol and Substance Abuse Among Schizophrenic Patients Presenting to an Emergency Psychiatric Service." *Journal of Nervous and Mental Disease*, 1989, *177*, 400–407.

Bassuk, E. L., Rubin, L., and Lauriat, A. "Is Homelessness a Mental Health Problem?" *American Journal of Psychiatry*, 1984, *141*, 1546–1550.

Benda, B. B., and Datallo, P. "Homelessness: Consequence of a Crisis or a Long-Term Process?" *Hospital and Community Psychiatry*, 1988, *39*, 884–886.

Bergman, H. C., and Harris, M. "Substance Use Among Young Adult Chronic Patients." *Psychosocial Rehabilitation Journal*, 1985, *9*, 49–54.

Berkson, J. "Limitations of the Application of Four-Fold Tables to Hospital Data." *Biometric Bulletin*, 1946, *2*, 47–53.

Bowers, M. B., and Swigar, M. E. "Vulnerability to Psychosis Associated with Hallucinogen Use." *Psychiatry Research*, 1983, *9*, 91–97.

Boyd, J. H., Burke, J. D., Gruenberg, E., and others. "Exclusion Criteria of DSM-III: A Study of Co-Occurrence of Hierarchy-Free Syndromes." *Archives of General Psychiatry*, 1984, *41*, 983–989.

Breakey, W. R., Goodell, H., Lorenz, P. C., and McHugh, P. R. "Hallucinogenic Drugs as Precipitants of Schizophrenia." *Psychological Medicine*, 1974, *4*, 255–261.

Carey, M. P., Carey, K. B., and Meisler, A. W. "Psychiatric Symptoms in Mentally Ill Chemical Abusers." *Journal of Nervous and Mental Disease*, in press.

Caton, C.L.M. "The New Chronic Patient and the System of Community Care." *Hospital and Community Psychiatry*, 1981, *32*, 475–478.

Caton, C.L.M., Gralnick, A., Bender, S., and Simon, R. "Young Chronic Patients and Substance Abuse." *Hospital and Community Psychiatry*, 1989, *40*, 1037–1040.

Dixon, L., Haas, G., Weiden, P., Sweeney, J., and Frances, A. "Acute Effects of Drug Abuse in Schizophrenic Patients: Clinical Observations and Patients' Self-Reports." *Schizophrenia Bulletin*, 1990, *16*, 69–79.

Drake, R. E., Osher, F. C., and Wallach, M. A. "Alcohol Use and Abuse in Schizophrenia: A Prospective Community Study." *Journal of Nervous and Mental Disease*, 1989, *177*, 408–414.

Drake, R. E., Teague, G. B., and Warren, S. R. "New Hampshire's Dual Diagnosis Program for People with Severe Mental Illness and Substance Abuse." *Addiction and Recovery*, 1990, *10*, 35–39.

Drake, R. E., and Wallach, M. A. "Substance Abuse Among the Chronic Mentally Ill." *Hospital and Community Psychiatry*, 1989, *40*, 1041–1046.

Drake, R. E., Wallach, M. A., Teague, G. B., Freeman, D. H., Paskus, T. S., and Clark, T. A. "Housing Instability and Homelessness Among Rural Schizophrenic Patients." *American Journal of Psychiatry*, in press.

Galanter, M., Castaneda, R., and Ferman, J. "Substance Abuse Among General Psychiatric Patients: Place of Presentation, Diagnosis, and Treatment." *American Journal of Alcohol Abuse*, 1988, *14*, 211-235.

Group for the Advancement of Psychiatry. *Interactive Fit: A Guide to Nonpsychotic Chronic Patients*. Report no. 121. New York: Brunner/Mazel, 1987.

Hellerstein, D. J., and Meehan, B. "Outpatient Group Therapy for Schizophrenic Substance Abusers." *American Journal of Psychiatry*, 1987, *144*, 1337-1339.

Kesselman, M. S., Solomon, J., Beaudett, M., and Thornton, B. "Alcoholism and Schizophrenia." In J. Solomon (ed.), *Alcoholism and Clinical Psychiatry*. New York: Plenum 1982.

Kofoed, L., Kania, J., Walsh, T., and Atkinson, R. M. "Outpatient Treatment of Patients with Substance Abuse and Co-Existing Psychiatric Disorders." *American Journal of Psychiatry*, 1986, *143*, 867-872.

Kroll, J., Carey, K., Hagedorn, D., Fire Dog, P., and Benavides, E. "A Survey of Homeless Adults in Urban Emergency Shelters." *Hospital and Community Psychiatry*, 1986, *37*, 283-286.

Lamb, H. R. "Young Adult Chronic Patients: The New Drifters." *Hospital and Community Psychiatry*, 1982, *33*, 465-468.

Lamb, H. R. (ed.). *The Homeless Mentally Ill: A Task Force Report of the American Psychiatric Association*. Washington, D.C.: American Psychiatric Press, 1984.

Lamb, H. R., and Grant, R. W. "The Mentally Ill in an Urban County Jail." *Archives of General Psychiatry*, 1982, *39*, 17-22.

Lehmann, A. F., Myers, C. P., and Corty, E. "Assessment and Classification of Patients with Psychiatric and Substance Abuse Syndromes." *Hospital and Community Psychiatry*, 1989, *40*, 1019-1025.

Lieberman, J. A., and Bowers, M. "Substance Abuse Comorbidity in Schizophrenia." *Schizophrenia Bulletin*, 1990, *16*, 29-30.

McCarrick, A. K., Manderscheid, R. W., and Bertolucci, D. E. "Correlates of Acting-Out Behaviors Among Young Adult Chronic Patients." *Hospital and Community Psychiatry*, 1985, *44*, 259-261.

McLellan, A. T., Woody, G. E., and O'Brien, C. P. "Development of Psychiatric Illness in Drug Abusers: Possible Role of Drug Preference." *New England Journal of Medicine*, 1979, *301*, 1310-1314.

Minkoff, K. "Beyond Deinstitutionalization: A New Ideology for the Postinstitutional Era." *Hospital and Community Psychiatry*, 1987, *38*, 945-950.

Minkoff, K. "An Integrated Treatment Model for Dual Diagnosis of Psychosis and Addiction." *Hospital and Community Psychiatry*, 1989, *40*, 1031-1036.

National Institute on Drug Abuse. *National Household Survey on Drug Abuse: Population Estimates 1985*. Department of Health and Human Services publication no. (ADM) 87-1539. Rockville, Md.: National Institute on Drug Abuse, 1987.

Noordsy, D. L., Drake, R. E., Teague, G. B., Osher, F. C., Hurlbut, S. C., Beaudett, M. S., and Paskus, T. S. "Subjective Experiences Related to Alcohol Use Among Schizophrenics." *Journal of Nervous and Mental Disease*, in press.

Osher, F. C., Drake, R. E., Noordsy, D. L., Teague, G. B., Hurlbut, S. C., Beaudett, M. S., and Paskus, T. S. "Correlates of Alcohol Abuse Among Rural Schizophrenic Patients." Unpublished manuscript, New Hampshire-Dartmouth Psychiatric Research Center, 1991.

Osher, F. C., and Kofoed, L. L. "Treatment of Patients with Psychiatric and Psychoactive Substance Abuse Disorders." *Hospital and Community Psychiatry*, 1989, *40*, 1025-1030.

Pepper, B., Kirshner, M. C., and Ryglewicz, H. "The Young Adult Chronic Patient: Overview of a Population." *Hospital and Community Psychiatry,* 1981, *32,* 463-469.

Regier, D. A., and Burke, J. D. "Psychiatric Disorders in the Community: The Epidemiologic Catchment Area Study." In R. E. Hales and A. J. Frances (eds.), *American Psychiatric Association Annual Review.* Vol. 6. Washington, D.C.: American Psychiatric Press, 1987.

Regier, D. A., Farmer, M. E., Rae, D. S., Locke, B. Z., Keith, S. J., Judd, L. L., and Goodwin, F. K. "Comorbidity of Mental Disorders with Alcohol and Other Drug Abuse." *Journal of the American Medical Association,* 1990, *264,* 2511-2518.

Regier, D. A., Myers, J. K., Kramer, M., and others. "The NIMH Epidemiologic Catchment Area Program: Historical Context, Major Objectives, and Study Population Characteristics." *Archives of General Psychiatry,* 1984, *41,* 934-941.

Richardson, M. A., Craig, T. J., and Haugland, G. "Treatment Patterns of Young Chronic Schizophrenic Patients in the Era of Deinstitutionalization." *Psychiatric Quarterly,* 1985, *57,* 104-110.

Ridgely, M. S., Goldman, H. H., and Talbott, J. A. *Chronic Mentally Ill Young Adults with Substance Abuse Problems: A Review of the Literature and Creation of a Research Agenda.* Baltimore: Mental Health Policy Studies, University of Maryland School of Medicine, 1986.

Ridgely, M. S., Osher, F. C., and Talbott, J. A. *Chronic Mentally Ill Young Adults with Substance Abuse Problems: Treatment and Training Issues.* Baltimore: Mental Health Policy Studies, University of Maryland School of Medicine, 1987.

Robbins, E., Stern, M., Robbins, L., and others. "Unwelcome Patients: Where Can They Find Asylum?" *Hospital and Community Psychiatry,* 1978, *29,* 44-46.

Roth, D., and Bean, G. J. "New Perspectives on Homelessness: Findings from a State-Wide Epidemiological Study." *Hospital and Community Psychiatry,* 1986, *37,* 712-719.

Safer, D. "Substance Abuse by Young Adult Chronic Patients." *Hospital and Community Psychiatry,* 1987, *38,* 511-514.

Schneier, F. R., and Siris, S. G. "A Review of Psychoactive Substance Use and Abuse in Schizophrenia: Patterns of Drug Choice." *Journal of Nervous and Mental Disease,* 1987, *175,* 641-652.

Schutt, R. K., and Garrett, G. R. "Social Background, Residential Experience, and Health Problems of the Homeless." *Psychosocial Rehabilitation Journal,* 1988, *12,* 67-70.

Schwartz, S. R., and Goldfinger, S. M. "The New Chronic Patient: Clinical Characteristics of an Emerging Subgroup." *Hospital and Community Psychiatry,* 1981, *32,* 470-474.

Solomon, P. "Receipt of Aftercare Services by Problem Types: Psychiatric, Psychiatric/Substance Abuse, and Substance Abuse." *Psychiatric Quarterly,* 1986-87, *58,* 180-188.

Teague, G. B., Schwab, B., and Drake, R. E. *Evaluating Services for Young Adults with Dual Diagnoses of Severe Mental Illness and Substance Use Disorder.* Alexandria, Va.: National Association of State Mental Health Program Directors, 1990.

Turner, W. M., and Tsuang, M. T. "Impact of Substance Abuse on the Course and Outcome of Schizophrenia." *Schizophrenia Bulletin,* 1990, *16,* 87-95.

Yesavage, J. A., and Zarcone, V. "History of Drug Abuse and Dangerous Behavior in Inpatient Schizophrenics." *Journal of Clinical Psychiatry,* 1983, *44,* 259-261.

Robert E. Drake, M.D., Ph.D., is director of the New Hampshire–Dartmouth Psychiatric Research Center.

Peggy McLaughlin, M.S.W., J.D., is clinical coordinator of The Information Exchange.

Bert Pepper, M.D., is executive director of The Information Exchange.

Kenneth Minkoff, M.D., is chief of psychiatry at the Caulfield Center of Choate Health Systems.

Using an integrated theoretical framework, a continuous and comprehensive model system of care for dual diagnosis patients can be designed.

Program Components of a Comprehensive Integrated Care System for Serious Mentally Ill Patients with Substance Disorders

Kenneth Minkoff

During the last two decades, deinstitutionalization has been increasingly associated with the emergence of large numbers of individuals with concomitant substance disorders and severe, chronic psychiatric disorders. The breadth of this problem has been documented by numerous studies measuring the prevalence of substance abuse and substance dependence among chronically mentally ill patients. These studies have indicated a rate of substance abuse—variously defined and measured—of between 32 and 85 percent, and prevalence of substance dependence—again variously defined and measured—of between 15 and 40 percent (Pepper and others, 1981; Schwartz and Goldfinger, 1981; Alterman, 1985; Safer, 1987; Caton, Gralnick, Bender, and Simon, 1989; Drake, Osher, and Wallach, 1989). Similarly, ECA studies have demonstrated a markedly increased prevalence of severe psychiatric disorders, such as schizophrenia and bipolar disorder, among patients with substance dependence diagnoses (Regier and others, 1990).

Such large numbers of dual diagnosis patients have clearly created significant difficulties not only for individual clinicians and programs, but for entire systems of care—both for the addiction system and for the mental health system. Bachrach (1986-87) has written that these patients are frequently "system misfits"; they do not readily conform to established expectations within each system for obtaining access to care. Addiction programs and addiction clinicians are often ill-equipped to deal with addicted patients who present with psychotic symptoms and/or who require prescription of psychotropic medication, and mental health programs are often similarly ill-equipped to treat patients who require an abstinent environment and/or an intensive addiction recovery support system in which to address substance abuse or dependence. Development of integrated or hybrid programs has been proposed as a solution to this dilemma (Ridgely, Osher, and Talbott, 1987; Osher and Kofoed, 1989; Sciacca, 1987), but even where such programs exist they cannot adequately respond to either the diversity of dual diagnosis patients or to the sheer numbers of them within any given care system.

The literature on treatment of dual diagnosis patients has described specific clinical techniques (Kofoed, Kania, Walsh, and Atkinson, 1986; Evans and Sullivan, 1990; Osher and Kofoed, 1989) and individual hybrid treatment programs (Ridgely, Osher, and Talbott, 1987; Minkoff, 1989), but with rare exceptions (Drake and others, in this volume), it has not addressed the more complex problem of how to design a comprehensive care *system* to meet the needs of the dual diagnosis population as a whole. The purpose of this chapter is (1) to define specific issues that must be addressed in a comprehensive care system, (2) to describe an integrated theoretical framework for understanding dual diagnosis, and (3) to use this framework to develop a model system of care.

Issues in Designing an Integrated System

Addiction System Versus Mental Health System. As noted earlier, dual diagnosis patients appear with significant frequency in both systems. Consequently, a comprehensive care network for dual diagnosis patients must incorporate and integrate elements of both systems. In a review of selected treatment programs for dual diagnosis patients nationwide, Ridgely, Osher, and Talbott (1987, p. 11) observe that "the fields of mental health and substance abuse have different foci, different philosophies, and a history of contentious behavior toward one another." These philosophical differences include conflicts concerning the use of medication, the quasi-religious nature of twelve-step programs, the predominant role of addiction counselors (as opposed to psychiatrists, psychologists, and social workers) in many addiction programs, the issue of which diagnosis should be primary, and so on. In addition, these philosophical differences are reinforced, in most states, by structural separation of addiction services and mental health services into distinct departments with separate and often competing hierarchies, funding mechanisms, methods for delivering care, patterns of regionalization of services, and organizational cultures (Ridgely, Goldman, and Willenbring, 1990). Separation of administrative authority for mental health and substance abuse services exists in twenty-one of fifty-five states and territories (Ridgely, Goldman, and Willenbring, 1990). This separation is reinforced by the division of ADAMHA into three separate institutions (NIMH, NIAAA, and NIDA) at the federal level (Ridgely, Goldman, and Willenbring, 1990).

As a result, any workable plan for providing comprehensive services to dual diagnosis patients must either completely reorganize the structure of state government or develop an integrated philosophical perspective that permits each system or department to define a meaningful role in addressing the problem and to identify *focused* areas of intersystem collaboration (Illinois Department of Mental Health and Developmental Disabilities, 1990).

Integrated Treatment Versus Parallel or Sequential Treatment. Any comprehensive care system for dual diagnosis patients must balance reliance on hybrid programs that provide simultaneous addiction and psychiatric treatment (integrated treatment) with utilization of diverse generic program elements that provide individual episodes of psychiatric or addiction treatment to dual diagnosis patients (parallel or sequential treatment). Later in this volume, Kline and colleagues compare the benefits of integrated treatment and parallel treatment in a dually diagnosed homeless mentally ill population. Potential benefits of hybrid treatment include the opportunity to provide simultaneous treatment under one supervisory umbrella, with a unified case management perspective, by dually trained clinicians, in a setting specifically designed to accommodate *both* disorders. A significant problem with this model, however, is the difficulty of developing sufficient numbers and varieties of hybrid programs to accommodate both the numbers of dual diagnosis patients and the variations in their diagnoses, levels of acuity, levels of disability, and degree of motivation.

Parallel treatment, by contrast, allows for utilization of existing treatment resources (with modification) in both care systems. It can have more flexibility in permitting clients to move through the care systems as they progress and to participate in more "normalizing" types of addiction treatment (such as Alcoholics Anonymous and Narcotics Anonymous). Many patients, particularly those who are homeless, may find it easier to engage with services that do not address mental illness (Kline, Harris, Bebout, and Drake, in this volume); others will engage more readily in services that do not address substance abuse. The major limitation of parallel treatment, however, is the enormous burden placed on case managers—and clients— to maintain continuity through multiple episodes of treatment in diverse programs in distinct systems of care. Suitable programs also need to be located for many clients who do not readily fit into existing program models.

Care Versus Confrontation. Traditionally, the mental health system— in particular, the community support system model (Stroul, 1989)—has organized services according to principles of "case management": providing care and support for individuals with various levels of psychiatric disability. The orientation has been to identify individual limitations and deficits, and then assertively to provide clients *what they need*. Traditional twelve-step addiction programs, by contrast, emphasize individual responsibility and motivation rather than disability. To achieve sobriety, patients must be confronted—in a caring way—by the negative consequences of their addiction in order to generate motivation for recovery. They must then take responsibility for accepting help. The orientation of twelve-step programs, therefore, is to identify the help that is available and then provide people what they are *willing to ask for*. In the mental health system, if a patient refuses help, the case manager takes responsibility and attempts to minimize the negative consequences to the patient. In the addiction system, if a patient refuses help, the clinician is encouraged to "detach" and to allow the patient to bear the responsibility for the negative consequences of his or her refusal.

Clearly, any system of care for dual diagnosis patients must balance care and support for patients' disabilities with empathic confrontation of patients with responsibility for their own recovery. Further, since dual diagnosis patients vary in their levels of disability and motivation, the care system must offer a range of programs that combine care and detachment in various proportions for different patient populations.

Abstinence-Oriented Versus Abstinence-Mandated Programs. A common controversy in programs for dually diagnosed patients is whether to mandate abstinence as a precondition of participation or to encourage abstinence as a goal. Traditional twelve-step programs of addiction treatment clearly indicate that if abstinence is not mandated, the treatment program loses both its credibility and its effectiveness. On the other hand, numerous authors (Kofoed, Kania, Walsh, and Atkinson, 1986; Sciacca, 1987; Osher and Kofoed, 1989) have emphasized that, for the dually diagnosed patient, requiring abstinence at the outset discourages or prevents engagement in treatment. Thus, many hybrid dual diagnosis programs define abstinence as a *goal,* and encourage patients to make incremental steps toward that goal through gradual reduction in the amount and frequency of substance use. Such programs may be unable, however, to provide for clients who require a completely abstinent environment in order to initiate or maintain sobriety.

A comprehensive care system for dual diagnosis patients, therefore, may require a *combination* of abstinence-mandated and abstinence-oriented programs, with clear guidelines defining the respective roles of each.

Deinstitutionalization Versus Recovery and Rehabilitation. One issue that faces any care system for the chronically mentally ill is the system's broad definition of its overall mission and philosophy. For several decades, the treatment of the chronically mentally ill has been dominated by the *deinstitutionalization ideology* (Minkoff, 1987). This defines "good care" as care outside of state institutions in community settings, in which the goal is always to encourage the client to utilize the "least restrictive" and least intensive alternative, and in which success is measured by reduction in state hospital census and admissions.

Addiction treatment, on the other hand, has, in the twelve-step model, been dominated by a philosophy of *recovery*, in which neither locus of care nor short-term morbidity is as significant as the long-term outcome goals of persistent sobriety and growing serenity, self-acceptance, and inner peace. In the recovery model, patients are often encouraged to ask for *more* help in the short run—in more intensive and restrictive settings (inpatient rehabilitation programs, halfway houses, therapeutic communities)—to bring about a more successful long-term outcome.

In recent years, the recovery/rehabilitation ideology has begun to supplant the deinstitutionalization ideology in the treatment of the chronically mentally ill (Harding and others, 1987; Minkoff, 1987), and the role of the patient in taking responsibility for long-term recovery from psychosis has been clarified (Strauss and others, 1987). Thus, for the chronically mentally ill (and, by extension, for the dually diagnosed population), locus of care is becoming less important than maximizing long-term recovery. This implies that extended public hospitalization for dually diagnosed patients may sometimes be appropriate (Group for the Advancement of Psychiatry, 1982). It also means that in some situations, progression to a less restrictive alternative may be made conditional on a patient's taking responsibility for "working a program of recovery" for *both* illnesses.

In designing a system of care for dual diagnosis patients, therefore, the goal of maximizing recovery must be primary, but also must be integrated with the goal of minimizing reliance on restrictive institutions. It cannot be expected or assumed, however, that pushing clients into less restrictive settings with more freedom will always enhance the recovery process.

The purpose of this chapter is to describe a comprehensive continuous and integrated system of care for dual diagnosis patients that addresses the five issues discussed earlier. To design this system, we need to integrate the simultaneous treatment of mental illness and addiction within a unified conceptual framework.

Integrated Conceptual Framework for Dual Diagnosis

Minkoff (1989) has described an integrated conceptual framework for the treatment of dual diagnosis of serious mental illness and substance dependence in a general hospital inpatient unit. The elements of this conceptual framework are as follows:

1. Chronic psychotic disorders and substance dependence are both viewed as examples of chronic mental illness, with many common characteristics (biological etiology, hereditability, chronicity, incurability, treatability, potential for relapse and deterioration, denial, and associated shame and guilt), despite distinctive differences in symptomatology.

2. Each illness can fit into a disease-and-recovery model for assessment and treatment, where the goal of treatment is to stabilize acute symptoms and then *engage the person* who has the disease to participate in a long-term program of maintenance, rehabilitation, and recovery.

3. Regardless of order of onset, each illness is considered *primary.* Further, although each illness can exacerbate the symptoms of and interfere with the treatment of the other, the severity and level of disability associated with each illness is regarded as essentially *independent* of the severity and level of disability associated with the other. Consequently, patients who have dual diagnoses must receive specific and concurrent treatments for *both* primary diagnoses. For mental illness, this treatment generally involves maintenance medication and rehabilitation programming; for addiction, this treatment involves detoxification, stabilization within a support system such as AA, and participation in a recovery program (for example, twelve steps, residential therapeutic community).

4. Both illnesses can be regarded as having *parallel* phases of treatment and recovery. According to Minkoff (1989), those phases include acute stabilization, engagement in treatment, prolonged stabilization/maintenance, and rehabilitation/recovery. Osher and Kofoed (1989) have further subdivided the engagement phase into engagement, persuasion, and active treatment; prolonged stabilization is the intended outcome of active treatment.

5. Although, in dual diagnosis patients, progress in recovery for each diagnosis is *affected* by progress in recovery for the other, the recovery processes commonly proceed independently. In particular, progress in recovery may depend on patient motivation, and patient motivation for treatment of each illness may vary. Thus, patients may be engaged in active treatment to maintain stabilization of psychosis, while still refusing treatment for stabilization of substance abuse. Alternatively, patients may be actively sober in AA, yet deny the need for psychotropic medication for mental illness (Minkoff, 1989).

This conceptual framework has the following implications for designing a dual diagnosis system of care:

Each care system must include program elements that meet the needs of patients in *each phase of recovery for each illness.* Thus, some programs may provide active treatment for one illness and maintenance for the other. There must, for example, be programs for acute detoxification of stable mentally ill individuals, as well as programs for patients who require simultaneous detoxification and stabilization of psychosis; programs for beginning the process of engagement and persuasion to involve stable mentally ill patients in substance abuse treatment, and programs for stable mentally ill patients who want and need active abstinence-mandated addiction treatment; and so on.

Each care system must include program elements that address various levels of *severity* and *disability* in each illness in each phase of recovery. For example, there may be a range of community residence programs that includes a residence appropriate for severely disabled mentally ill people with substance problems that are amenable to outpatient treatment, a residence appropriate for highly functioning mentally ill individuals who are severely addicted and need an abstinent environment to maintain sobriety, and a residence for people who are severely ill with both illnesses. (All three models are described in other chapters in this volume.)

Each system of care must include program elements suitable for clients who have various levels of *motivation* for assuming responsibility for their recovery. The system must provide adequate levels of care for those who are disabled but unmotivated, while creating systemwide incentives for clients to progress to programs that are more desirable but also more demanding.

Some dual diagnosis programs will ideally be extensions of existing generic programs within either the addiction or mental health system into which dual diagnosis patients are integrated. Others will be specific hybrid programs that serve *only* dually diagnosed patients. The illness being treated most actively, the phase of treatment, and the patients' level of severity, disability, and motivation will determine within which system a program is best located and whether the program should be generic or specific.

Development of a Model System of Care

Bachrach (1986) has identified continuity and comprehensiveness as key elements in the design of a model system of care. I will discuss each element separately.

Continuity. Within any comprehensive array of services, the care system needs to provide for continuity of treatment between programs, as well as continuity over time. This is a particular problem for dual diagnosis patients, who often experience "ping-pong treatment" (Ridgely, Goldman, and Willenbring, 1990) as they bounce back and forth between two distinct care systems. Although involvement of patients in ongoing hybrid programs facilitates continuity of care, most patients will still need to be involved with multiple programs in different phases of treatment throughout their long-term course. Consequently, development of an integrated dual diagnosis case management program is a necessary ingredient in creating a dual diagnosis care system.

Ideally, dual diagnosis case management involves both the addiction system and the mental health system. Although dual diagnosis case management programs have been created entirely within the mental health system utilizing teams of dually trained clinicians (Harris and Bergman, 1987), the most recent models have been developed through statewide collaborations between mental health and substance abuse authorities

(Drake, Teague, and Warren, 1990; Illinois Department of Mental Health and Developmental Disabilities, 1990). In both New Hampshire and Illinois, in fact, the implementation of a collaborative dual diagnosis case management program has been the necessary first step in pulling together diverse program components to provide individual patients with a beginning comprehensive system of care.

Comprehensiveness. As we have discussed, a comprehensive care system for dual diagnosis patients will include programs within both the addiction system and the mental health system, as well as some collaborative programs. Integrated treatment programs will be one type of program element within a broad parallel treatment model that incorporates a range of hybrid and generic programs. Programs will be designed to focus on different phases of treatment and different levels of motivation, severity, and disability related to each illness, and will include both abstinence-oriented and abstinence-mandated programs. Programs will be defined by the level of care and support provided, and the level of patient responsibility expected, for treatment of each illness.

One principle I have used in developing this model is to build on existing systems and programs wherever possible, and to minimize the extent to which additional specialized dual diagnosis programs must be developed. This approach is not only less costly, it reflects the reality that dual diagnosis is so prevalent that it must be addressed (to some extent) as part of *routine* treatment in either care system.

Unfortunately, in some states existing care systems for single diagnosis patients are sadly deficient. In such states, more creative solutions for dual diagnosis patients will be necessary. For example, in a state that has little public funding available for alcohol and drug treatment, the mental health system may have to take a leadership role in developing generic addiction detoxification or rehabilitation services as a resource for dually diagnosed clients.

I will now describe the specific programs in this model for each phase of treatment of each illness.

Acute Stabilization. For dual diagnosis patients, acute stabilization of psychiatric symptoms generally occurs within the mental health system, usually in an acute psychiatric inpatient unit. Patients with less severe symptoms may be treated in outpatient or day hospital settings, while patients with the most severe disturbances will require access to a locked facility. Ries (1990) has observed that severe behavioral symptoms (psychosis, violence, suicidality) may require acute psychiatric inpatient treatment, even when such symptoms are solely related to substance abuse. To treat patients with coexisting substance disorders, the traditional acute psychiatric unit needs to develop the following capabilities: (1) capacity to provide detoxification for substance-dependent patients, (2) protocols to identify substance abuse and dependence disorders, (3) capacity to initiate education and engagement regarding substance use, and (4) referral linkages to programs that can continue the process of engagement for both substance disorders and psychiatric disorders.

Acute stabilization of addiction symptoms within the addiction system usually occurs in a detoxification program. Less severely ill addiction patients can discontinue use without detoxification, or receive detoxification on an outpatient basis: access to a methadone maintenance program may provide outpatient acute stabilization for narcotic addicts. More severely substance-dependent individuals who are endangering themselves or others and who are unable to accept help, yet do not have acute psychiatric symptoms, may require involuntary detoxification.

With regard to dual diagnosis patients, the generic detoxification programs listed earlier are potentially appropriate for individuals with (1) stable psychotic mental illness without severe residual symptoms, (2) personality disorders without severe behavioral disturbance, or (3) a range of anxiety, depressive, and post-traumatic stress disorders. To accommodate such patients, the following capacities can be developed: (1) ability to provide medication other than for detoxification (stable regimen only) and to support its continued use if indicated; (2) protocols for assessment of coexisting psychiatric disorder, and for ensuring sufficient psychiatric stability to permit admission; (3) availability of psychiatric consultation for difficult cases; and (4) referral linkage to both acute and maintenance psychiatric programs and to engagement programs for substance dependence.

In some areas, specialized detoxification programs have been developed collaboratively to address the needs of patients who have behavioral disturbances *while intoxicated* that are too severe for a standard detoxification program, but that resolve without other specific intervention (for example, personality-disordered alcoholics who are suicidal when drunk) and therefore do not require psychiatric hospitalization.

Engagement, Education, and Persuasion

For most dual diagnosis patients, engagement in treatment for major mental illness generally occurs within the mental health system, most commonly in an inpatient unit following acute stabilization. The most severely psychotic patients may require involuntary treatment and involuntary medication, and, occasionally, prolonged hospitalization in a public mental hospital. By contrast, many patients, particularly homeless mentally ill individuals, are engaged through community-based intensive case management and outreach programs (Harris and Bergman, 1987; Kline, Harris, Bebout, and Drake, in this volume). As noted earlier, such programs must also have the capacity to initiate education and engagement regarding coexisting substance disorders. In addition, they should either provide or have referral linkages to programs that provide ongoing stabilization for mental illness and continuing engagement and persuasion efforts regarding substance abuse (see below).

For most addiction patients, engagement in treatment for substance abuse in the addiction system occurs during the "rehabilitation" phase of inpatient addiction treatment. With the advent of managed care, many programs are also developing intensive day and evening treatment models (Batten and others, 1989). Such programs mandate abstinence as a condition of participation, and can be suitable for *motivated* dual diagnosis patients who have (1) stable psychotic mental illness without severe residual symptoms; (2) personality disorders without severe behavioral disturbance; or (3) a range of coexisting anxiety, depressive, and post-traumatic stress disorders. To accommodate such patients, the capacities listed earlier for detoxification programs must be available, as well as referrals to long-term addiction support programs such as outpatient AA and residential settings.

Integrated addiction and psychiatry units, such as that described by Minkoff (1989), can be ideal settings to initiate engagement in treatment for both illnesses simultaneously, particularly for patients whose psychiatric symptoms are not completely stabilized or are more severe at baseline. Such a program can also provide more in-depth assessment of difficult "dual diagnostic dilemmas." In systems where such an integrated program is not available, simultaneous parallel treatment in neighboring collaborative units can sometimes work nearly as well. Less beneficial is sequential treatment in noncollaborative programs (Ries, 1990; Ridgely, Goldman, and Willenbring, 1990).

Engagement in treatment for substance *abuse* (as distinct from dependence) for mentally ill patients—and for all substance disorders for more severely disabled mentally ill patients—generally begins in the setting in which the patient is receiving treatment for ongoing stabilization of the mental illness.

Ongoing Stabilization and Rehabilitation

Within the mental health system, ongoing stabilization, treatment, and rehabilitation for dually diagnosed patients occur in a range of outpatient, day treatment, and residential settings, depending on the level of severity of patients' disabilities and, to a lesser extent, on their willingness to comply with treatment requirements. The most severely ill and least motivated require long-term residential treatment and self-contained day programming in public mental hospitals; those with illnesses of moderate severity live in supervised residences or in the care of family members and participate in various types of day programming; and those with the least severe illnesses may live independently and participate in standard outpatient treatment. Homeless patients may be engaged in ongoing case management and day programming even prior to receiving housing (Harris and Bergman, 1987).

Dual diagnosis patients engaged in mental health treatment in these settings are frequently unwilling either to recognize or to seek treatment for their coexisting substance disorders. Consequently, each of these settings needs to develop integrated or hybrid program models that address substance abuse and substance dependence within the setting itself.

Several such models are described in the literature (Osher and Kofoed, 1989; Sciacca, 1987), and in later chapters in this volume. Common characteristics of these programs in the *outpatient* setting are as follows:

1. Abstinence is a goal, not a requirement.
2. Patients with substance abuse and substance dependence are treated together.
3. Group models, with either staff or peer leaders, are fundamental.
4. Patients progress from (a) low-level education or "persuasion" groups, in which patients have high denial and low motivation, to (b) "active treatment" groups, in which they are more motivated to consider abstinence and are willing to accept more confrontation, to (c) abstinence support groups, in which they have mostly committed to abstinence and help each other to learn new skills to attain or maintain sobriety (Osher and Kofoed, 1989).
5. Involvement of available family members is recommended.

Residential programming has similar goals, and generally can incorporate a variety of residential models:

a. Integrating dual diagnosis patients into a generic mental health residence and providing substance abuse treatment as part of a day program.
b. Creating a dual diagnosis residence with abstinence as a goal, and with on-site dual diagnosis groups.
c. Developing a sober residence for *motivated* patients who require residential support, in which abstinence is mandated, or at least expected, and in which abstinence-support programming is built in.

Note that these distinctions can even be created within subdivisions of a state hospital.

Regardless of the type of substance programming offered, each program must define the level of substance-related problem behavior that cannot be tolerated within the program (for example, obvious intoxication, belligerence, selling or using drugs on premises, and so on) and develop a clear set of policies that determine the behavioral consequences for violations (Sciacca, in this volume). Such policies are not punitive, but rather provide necessary protection from drugs and alcohol, safety for other program participants, and leverage to encourage offending patients to accept more intensive substance dependence treatment, perhaps in an inpatient addiction unit. Consequences are only valid if they can be enforced, and provision *must* be made in the care system for patients who are suspended or discharged from day or residential programs due to persistent out-of-control substance involvement. In many systems, this will require making state hospitals available (deinstitutionalization ideology notwithstanding) for severely psychiatrically disabled actively addicted and unmotivated patients who otherwise might become homeless. In some locations, as an alternative, "wet" residential programs have been developed, where almost any amount of substance abuse can be tolerated (Blankertz and White, 1990).

Within the addiction system, extended support to maintain sobriety for severely addicted patients is generally available through a network of halfway houses (three to twelve months), therapeutic communities (twelve to twenty-four months), and sober houses (long-term), all of which are abstinence programs. Such programs are appropriate for motivated dual diagnosis patients who are otherwise capable of independent living, have reasonable social skills, and meet the diagnostic criteria listed earlier. These programs need to provide specialized training to staff in assessment and treatment of psychiatric disorders, and permit patients to self-administer stable regimens of nonaddictive medications. Psychiatric consultation is essential, and is best provided through linkage with an affiliated mental health provider that assumes concurrent and ongoing responsibility for the psychiatric treatment of these patients. In addition, such programs must provide linkage to ongoing outpatient *addiction* treatment, including individual, group, and family counseling, as well as twelve-step programs.

Traditional twelve-step programs in the addiction system are a valuable component of the ongoing addiction support system for dual diagnosis patients (Kofoed, Kania, Walsh, and Atkinson, 1986), particularly for patients who receive "special preparation" for selecting suitable groups and learning how to use the program properly (Ridgely, Osher, and Talbott, 1987; Minkoff, 1989). Even state hospital patients with severe psychiatric disabilities have been able to use twelve-step program attendance as an adjunctive support in maintaining sobriety.

Finally, collaborative or integrated programs to support ongoing stabilization and recovery can be developed in either system. Residences that provide a therapeutic community environment for treatment of addiction along with an infusion of psychiatric services for treatment of mental illness have emerged in the addiction system (McLaughlin and Pepper, in this volume), and traditional psychiatric residences that mandate sobriety with an intense addiction treatment focus have emerged in the mental health system. Often, these programs are cofunded or cosponsored by federal, state, or local mental health and addiction treatment authorities. Similarly, twelve-step programs specifically for dual diagnosis patients have emerged under the auspices of AA ("Double Trouble" meetings), and where such meetings do not exist, dual diagnosis peer-support groups using twelve-step principles can be developed in the mental health system.

Conclusion

I have described the dilemmas involved in dual diagnosis treatment and used a unified conceptual framework to design a model of a comprehensive, continuous, and integrated system of care for dual diagnosis patients. This model can be used by (1) system planners, to identify gaps that can be addressed by new program initiatives or by additional training resources; (2) program managers, to identify the role of each program within the total system and how to improve the program's capacity to treat dual diagnosis patients; and (3) individual case managers, to assess the capacities of their own system in relation to the needs of individual clients. Although the model contains generic as well as hybrid treatment programs, more successful systems will be characterized by better-developed case management and a greater number and variety of hybrid or integrated programs.

References

Alterman, A. I. "Substance Abuse in Psychiatric Patients." In A. I. Alterman (ed.), *Substance Abuse and Psychopathology.* New York: Plenum, 1985.

Bachrach, L. L. "The Challenge of Service Planning for Chronic Mental Patients." *Community Mental Health Journal,* 1986, *22,* 170-174.

Bachrach, L. L. "The Context of Care for the Chronic Mental Patient with Substance Abuse." *Psychiatric Quarterly,* 1986-87, *58,* 3-14.

Batten, H. L., Bachman, S., Higgins, R., Manzik, N., Minkoff, K., and Parham, C. "Implementation Issues in Addictions Day Treatment." *Hospital and Health Services Administration,* 1989, *34* (3), 427-439.

Blankertz, L., and White, K. K. "Implementation of a Rehabilitation Program for Dually Diagnosed Homeless." *Alcoholism Treatment Quarterly,* 1990, *7,* 149-164.

Caton, C.L.M., Gralnick, A., Bender, S., and Simon, R. "Young Chronic Patients and Substance Abuse." *Hospital and Community Psychiatry,* 1989, *40* (10), 1037-1040.

Drake, R. E., Osher, F. C., and Wallach, M. A. "Alcohol Use and Abuse in Schizophrenia: A Prospective Community Study." *Journal of Nervous and Mental Disease,* 1989, *177,* 408-414.

Drake, R. E., Teague, G. B., and Warren, S. R. "New Hampshire's Program for People Dually Diagnosed with Severe Mental Illness and Substance Use Disorders." *Addiction and Recovery,* 1990, *10,* 35-39.

Evans, K., and Sullivan, J. M. *Dual Diagnosis: Counseling the Mentally Ill Substance Abuser.* New York: Guilford Press, 1990.

Group for the Advancement of Psychiatry. *The Positive Aspects of Long-Term Hospitalization in the Public Sector for Chronic Psychiatric Patients.* Report no. 10. New York: Mental Health Materials Center, 1982.

Harding, C. M., Brooks, G. W., Ashikaga, T., and others. "The Vermont Longitudinal Study of Persons with Severe Mental Illness, II: Long-Term Outcome of Subjects Who Retrospectively Met DSM-III Criteria for Schizophrenia." *American Journal of Psychiatry,* 1987, *144,* 727–735.

Harris, M., and Bergman, H. "Case Management with the Chronically Mentally Ill: A Clinical Perspective." *American Journal of Orthopsychiatry,* 1987, *57* (2), 296–302.

Illinois Department of Mental Health and Developmental Disabilities. *Task Force Report for the Mentally Ill Substance Abuser.* Springfield: Illinois Department of Mental Health and Developmental Disabilities, 1990.

Kofoed, L., Kania, J., Walsh, T., and Atkinson, R. "Outpatient Treatment of Patients with Substance Abuse and Coexisting Psychiatric Disorders." *American Journal of Psychiatry,* 1986, *143,* 867–872.

Minkoff, K. "Beyond Deinstitutionalization: A New Ideology for the Postinstitutional Era." *Hospital and Community Psychiatry,* 1987, *38,* 945–950.

Minkoff, K. "An Integrated Treatment Model for Dual Diagnosis of Psychosis and Addiction." *Hospital and Community Psychiatry,* 1989, *40* (10), 1031–1036.

Osher, F. C., and Kofoed, L. L. "Treatment of Patients with Psychiatric and Psychoactive Substance Abuse Disorders." *Hospital and Community Psychiatry,* 1989, *40,* 1025–1030.

Pepper, B., Kirshner, M. C., and Ryglewicz, H. "The Young Adult Chronic Patient: Overview of a Population." *Hospital and Community Psychiatry,* 1981, *32,* 463–469.

Regier, D. A., Farmer, M. E., Rae, D. S., Locke, B. Z., Keith, S. J., Judd, L. L., and Goodwin, F. K. "Comorbidity of Mental Disorders with Alcohol and Other Drug Abuse." Results from the Epidemiologic Catchment Area (ECA) Study. *Journal of the American Medical Association,* 1990, *264* (19), 2511–2518.

Ridgely, M. S., Goldman, H. H., and Willenbring, M. "Barriers to the Care of Persons with Dual Diagnoses: Organizational and Financing Issues." *Schizophrenia Bulletin,* 1990, *16* (1), 123–132.

Ridgely, M. S., Osher, F. C., and Talbott, J. A. *Chronic Mentally Ill Young Adults with Substance Abuse Problems: Treatment and Training Issues.* Baltimore: Mental Health Policy Studies, School of Medicine, University of Maryland, 1987.

Ries, R. "Acute, Subacute, and Maintenance Treatment Phases for Dual Diagnosis Patients with the Public Mental Health Center." Unpublished manuscript, Department of Psychiatry, University of Washington, 1990.

Safer, D. J. "Substance Abuse by Young Adult Chronic Patients." *Hospital and Community Psychiatry,* 1987, *38,* 511–514.

Schwartz, S. R., and Goldfinger, S. M. "The New Chronic Patient: Clinical Characteristics of an Emerging Subgroup." *Hospital and Community Psychiatry,* 1981, *32,* 470–474.

Sciacca, K. "New Initiatives in the Treatment of the Chronic Patient with Alcohol/Substance Use Problems." *TIE Lines,* 1987, *4* (3), 5–6.

Strauss, J. S., Harding, C. M., Hafez, H., and others. "The Role of the Patient in Recovery from Psychosis." In J. S. Strauss, W. Boker, and H. D. Brenner (eds.), *Psychosocial Treatment of Schizophrenia.* Toronto, Canada: Huber, 1987.

Stroul, B. A. "Community Support Systems for Persons with Long-Term Mental Illness: A Conceptual Framework." *Psychosocial Rehabilitation Journal,* 1989, *12,* 9–26.

Kenneth Minkoff, M.D., is chief of psychiatric services at Choate Health Systems in Woburn, Mass., and medical director of the Caulfield Center, an integrated psychiatry and addiction hospital. He is on the clinical faculty of the Cambridge Hospital Department of Psychiatry of the Harvard Medical School.

While the state of the art in developing programs for severely mentally ill people with substance disorders is not well advanced, programs that show promise attend to a basic set of principles, providing or coordinating a core set of values.

Creating Integrated Programs for Severely Mentally Ill Persons with Substance Disorders

M. Susan Ridgely

The research literature on persons with severe mental disorders co-occurring with substance disorders (hereafter, dual diagnoses) suggests that substance abuse among those with severe mental disorders is a staggering service problem in both the public and private sectors. Recent reviews of the mental health and substance abuse literature (Ridgely, Goldman, and Talbott, 1986; Galanter, Castaneda, and Ferman, 1988) indicate that the problem of multiple illness or disabilities is the rule rather than the exception among persons seeking mental health and substance abuse treatment in the public sector, and that the problem has not been adequately addressed. Within the substance abuse literature, the co-occurrence of psychiatric symptomatology with substance abuse is associated with poor prognosis, regardless of substance abuse treatment modality (McLellan and others, 1983; Alterman, Erdlen, and Murphy, 1982). Mental health inter-

---

The terms *dual diagnosis* and *dual disorder* are used as descriptors for the co-occurrence of severe mental disorder and alcohol and other drug abuse disorders. Severe mental disorder refers to several mental disorders, including, primarily, schizophrenia, but also personality disorders and major affective disorders. Regardless of diagnosis, mental disorder is considered severe if it causes lasting disability and recurrent contact with the mental health system. Substance abuse refers to the use of alcohol and/or other drugs singly or in combination, resulting in a DSM-III-R diagnosis of substance abuse or substance dependence. Within this broad category of dually diagnosed are a diagnostically and functionally heterogeneous group of individuals with a variety of clinical needs.

NEW DIRECTIONS FOR MENTAL HEALTH SERVICES, no. 50, Summer 1991 © Jossey-Bass Inc., Publishers

ventions that do not attend to substance abuse problems produce poor outcomes for individuals with dual diagnoses (Safer, 1987; Hall, Popkin, and DeVaul, 1977; Cohen and Klein, 1974).

The literature colorfully describes the conflicts these persons generated for their caregivers. Their dysfunctional use of service systems is often accompanied by a dysfunctional style of contact with caregivers. One unfortunate consequence has been noted; it is clear that persons with dual disorders are often refused admission or discharged prematurely from care facilities in both sectors (Galanter, Castaneda, and Ferman, 1988; Ridgely, Goldman, and Willenbring, 1990).

Current approaches to treating persons with dual diagnoses emphasize the necessity of providing intensive and specific treatments for both illnesses concomitantly, combining the resources of mental health and substance abuse service systems (Ridgely, Osher, and Talbott, 1987; Lehmann, Myers, and Corty, 1989; Minkoff, 1989; Osher and Kofoed, 1989). However, coordinating a regimen of mental health and substance abuse services requires breaking out of the conventional categorical boundaries now separating the two service systems. Such organizational innovation and coordination rarely have been initiated. Consequently, individuals with dual diagnoses suffer from the excess burden of service systems designed for *single disabilities* that are as yet unable to accommodate their particular needs. Bachrach (1987) refers to this problem as an "externally imposed disability." Specific innovative programmatic interventions are necessary to overcome this "external disability."

Hybridization: Applying Existing Technology

One way of addressing the special needs of severely mentally ill persons with alcohol and other drug problems is to combine treatment for substance abuse with treatment for mental illness. This integrative approach, often referred to as *hybridization,* is favored by some in the field for both clinical and administrative reasons. First, clinically, hybridization permits titration of specific treatments for each disorder when both disorders are present. Second, hybridization eliminates the administrative burden of attempting to prescribe and deliver treatment to clients across multiple agencies and service systems. Often, people with dual diagnoses have been subject to so-called "ping-pong therapy." They are either bounced back and forth among agencies in each system or receive treatment in both systems, with each system unaware of the participation of the other.

Hybridization implies that dually diagnosed persons will receive their treatment for both disorders concomitantly within one setting rather than concurrently (or even serially) in different settings. This is possible because current programs for treatment of severely mentally ill persons and those for treatment of substance abuse share some common goals: (1) the recognition and control of problematic behavior, (2) the education of patients regarding their illness and the necessity of taking responsibility for its management, and (3) the provision of opportunities for positive community activities (educational, vocational, recreational) and relationships to foster stability and recovery. Hybridization is not the development of a whole new treatment technology for persons with dual disorders; rather, it is one method of applying existing psychiatric and substance abuse treatment technologies concomitantly.

Examples of Hybridized Treatment

Four programs may be used as examples of hybridized treatment programs for severely mentally ill persons with substance abuse disorders. These programs have been chosen because they illustrate the principles of integrated programming. The use of the term *example program* rather than *model program* is deliberate, though even the term *model program* does not necessarily imply that effectiveness has been demonstrated. We will move from inpatient to outpatient to psychosocial rehabilitation to community treatment in our brief review.

Caulfield Center. Minkoff (1989) reports on an integrated treatment program developed within the addiction unit at Caulfield Center, a community general hospital. This twenty-one-bed unit provides treatment for patients with a major psychosis and substance abuse or dependence. The integrated treatment program is based on "AA's 12-step disease-and-recovery model and the standard biopsychosocial model for treatment of serious psychiatric disorders." Under this integrated model, both addiction and major psychosis can be viewed as "chronic, biologic mental illnesses that can be treated through simultaneous application of parallel concepts from both the addiction and psychiatric models" (Minkoff, 1989, p. 1032). Specifically, these models emphasize stabilization of symptomatology as well as engaging the person in treatment and rehabilitation for each of the chronic illnesses (addiction and major mental illness). Parallel processes of recovery for both chronic illnesses are described, including: (1) acute stabilization, (2) engagement, (3) prolonged stabilization, and (4) rehabilitation.

Patients at Caulfield Center may be assigned to one of four specific treatment schedules, depending on their particular needs: addiction, psychiatric, mixed addiction (full addiction plus two days psychiatric per week), and mixed psychiatric (full psychiatric plus two days of addiction per week). The "mixed" treatment schedules allow for further differentiation of the dual diagnosis program, providing individualized tracks for patients in different phases of treatment.

Pilot Program for the Psychiatrically Impaired Substance Abuser (PISA). This is an outpatient program developed by the Portland (Oregon)

VA Medical Center's Alcohol and Drug Dependence Treatment Section. It is an open-ended treatment track offering residential and outpatient treatment using techniques drawn from both psychiatric and substance abuse treatment (Kofoed, Kania, Walsh, and Atkinson, 1986). To emphasize the importance of abstinence, the outpatient groups meet in the Alcohol and Drug Clinic, rather than the psychiatric clinic. Patients begin treatment by attending a weekly assessment group for six weeks. The initial focus is on stabilization of symptomatology, psychiatric medication management, and abstinence. In addition, the patients are educated about psychiatric and substance disorders and learn about the program. Once psychiatrically stable, patients are asked to begin taking disulfiram, going to AA, and developing goals for further treatment. Patients are expected to attend special one-and-a-half-hour weekly support groups and to continue with AA. Abstinence and medication compliance are monitored through breathalyzers, urine screens, and contacts with collaterals. Individual patients may receive other adjunctive therapies (individual, family counseling, day treatment, and so on) according to individual need (Kofoed, Kania, Walsh, and Atkinson, 1986).

The Gladstone Day Treatment Program. The Gladstone Day Treatment Program, part of Clackamas County (Oregon) Mental Health Program, is a psychosocial rehabilitation program for persons with severe mental disorders. (This program was visited in 1986 as a part of the federal Alcohol, Drug Abuse, and Mental Health Administration [ADAMHA] Project on Chronic Mentally Ill Young Adults with Substance Abuse Problems. [See Ridgely, Goldman, and Talbott, 1986; Ridgely, Osher, and Talbott, 1987.] Soon after our visit the director, Glenn Maynard, left Gladstone, and it is not clear that the program has continued as described here.) The program includes a social club, a vocational rehabilitation program, housing, and case management services. Substance abuse services are provided to clients of Gladstone through a cooperative staffing arrangement with the County Alcohol and Drug Programs. A substance abuse counselor works in tandem with the Gladstone staff on assessment and individualized treatment planning. In addition, the substance abuse counselor conducts two substance abuse groups within the Gladstone program. Initially, Gladstone clients are assessed and, if appropriate, enter an orientation group where the focus is on alcohol and drug education. The purpose of this staff-directed group is to break down denial and persuade the client about the need for substance abuse treatment. When clients are ready to commit to sobriety, they move to an active treatment group that is abstinence oriented and more peer-led. Clients are encouraged to take responsibility for their recovery and are given opportunities for vocational training and placement in independent apartments, as well as having access to social and recreational activities. Case managers reinforce the need for abstinence, as well as providing crisis intervention and concrete assistance with basic needs.

Community Connections. Finally, Kline, Harris, Bebout, and Drake (in this volume) have described the use of assertive community treatment in a program for homeless persons with dual diagnoses at Community Connections in Washington, D.C. This approach combines case management and in vivo clinical treatment according to a model developed and evaluated by Stein and Test in Madison, Wisconsin (Stein and Test, 1982; Willenbring, Ridgely, Stinchfield, and Rose, 1991). In the current adaptation at Community Connections, this powerful mental health treatment/case management intervention is combined with a full range of substance abuse services in-house that includes psychoeducation, individual counseling, and multilevel group work (Klein, Harris, Bebout, and Drake, in this volume). The integrated treatment process includes the following phases of treatment: (1) engagement, (2) persuasion, (3) active treatment, and (4) relapse prevention.

Principles of Integrated Programming

In reviewing the current literature on dual diagnosis treatment, and examining programs serving persons with dual diagnoses, including those discussed earlier, similarities in approach emerge. At this stage, absent treatment protocols verified by clinical trials, these similarities can serve as principles for the development of integrated treatment programs.

Most dual diagnosis treatment programs emphasize the need to address specific *phases* of treatment (Ridgely, Osher, and Talbott, 1987; Minkoff, 1989; Osher and Kofoed, 1989; Kline, Harris, Bebout, and Drake, in this volume). These phases involve essential service elements, to be provided by or directly affiliated with dual diagnosis programs, including interventions designed to: (1) engage clients in services; (2) motivate them to seek specific substance abuse treatment; (3) provide comprehensive assessment of alcohol, drug, and mental health problems; (4) provide concomitant treatment, including a core set of mental health and substance abuse treatment interventions; (5) provide or orchestrate relapse prevention or other aftercare interventions; and (6) develop linkages between the alcohol, drug, and mental health treatment systems. The following discussion will highlight some of the difficult issues programs face in each of these areas.

Engagement. The literature on severely mentally ill persons with substance abuse disorders stresses their crisis-oriented pattern of service utilization (Lamb, 1982; Bachrach, Talbott, and Meyerson, 1987) and the difficulty associated with establishing the trusting relationship necessary to get these persons into treatment. Engagement may be enhanced if program staff are able to help with crises in a concrete fashion (Lamb, 1982). Stein and Test (1982) also emphasize that engagement is not a one-time process, and highlight the necessity to *retain* clients in treatment as well as to attract them into treatment in the first place. An important concept in serving this population, therefore, is the concept of *interrupted treatment*. Rather than experiencing each break from treatment as a treatment failure (and a reason to refuse re-entry to the program), some dual diagnosis programs emphasize the fact that each entry represents an opportunity. Interrupted treatment allows for repeated contact over time, giving clinicians the opportunity to focus on small goals during each treatment episode, building on previous gains. Each contact becomes a window of opportunity (if clients can be persuaded to stay long enough) to foster further incremental breakdown of denial and minimization of both illnesses. Focusing in this way diminishes the need to either blame the staff or blame the client for a treatment "failure." While this may seem in conflict with the ideal of comprehensive, continuous treatment, it does recognize the reality of treating a very disabled clientele.

Engagement is also characterized by *approach/avoidance behavior*. Segal and Baumohl (1980), reviewing programming for homeless persons with severe mental illnesses, warn that lengthy intake procedures requiring the detailing of much personal information at the earliest stages may contribute to avoidance. They suggest these procedures be modified to require a minimum of information at the outset, with more information to be obtained during the process of engagement. Maximizing opportunities for informal interaction between staff and potential clients furthers the engagement process. For example, the social club atmosphere at psychosocial rehabilitation programs may be perceived as less threatening and less stigmatizing to some clients, and can allow empathic relationships to develop that may be a bridge into more intensive programming.

Engagement is a concern of the four example programs discussed earlier. Each has specifically addressed the need in its program protocols. For instance, Caulfield Center's inpatient program begins the engagement process during acute stabilization. The focus of engagement is on the development of a trusting, therapeutic relationship. Additionally, staff have found that a "judicious use of leverage" (such as court orders and family pressures) helps ensure that the patient will stay through the first stages of treatment (Minkoff, 1989). PISA and Gladstone use education about alcohol and drugs in a nonthreatening group environment as a means of initiating the treatment process. Community Connections, with its focus on homeless dually diagnosed persons, uses aggressive outreach and the development of a trusting relationship built on the provision of very basic services, such as assistance with housing, food, clothing, and other necessities. Individual counseling is emphasized, since many clients initially distrust providers and show, at best, ambivalence toward treatment (Kline, Harris, Bebout, and Drake, in this volume).

Persuasion. A related problem has to do with motivation for substance abuse treatment. Some programs are designed for clients who are motivated for treatment and have committed themselves to sobriety, in which case abstinence is a reasonable expectation early in the program. However, for many dually diagnosed persons, denial and minimization of substance abuse are particularly difficult to manage without the prior establishment of a trusting, therapeutic relationship. Requiring abstinence at the "front door" may make it impossible to engage them. Some programs, like Gladstone, have chosen to deal with this issue by not requiring total abstinence during the engagement process. Instead, staff proceed with alcohol and drug education and peer support activities, while giving the clients time and support to make their own decisions about when abstinence is a realistic goal. Rules are enforced, however, about use on the premises of the program facility in order to maintain the integrity of the program for use by other clients.

Some programs address the issue of motivation for substance abuse treatment by recognizing that most clients have concrete and immediate concerns, structuring initial program contacts around meeting these expressed needs. Such programs may include access to better housing, vocational training and job placement, and recreational activities as ways to engage and retain clients in treatment. These opportunities are tied, however, to staying in the program and working toward abstinence. Programs such as athletic clubs have used team sports as a way of enhancing peer group structures. Peer group influence is particularly strong in reinforcing the use of alcohol and other drugs and can be used in a similar way to reinforce abstinence.

Two of the above-mentioned example programs (PISA and Community Connections) identify *persuasion* as a separate phase of treatment. These two programs move beyond the goal of getting the individual to make a "genuine acknowledgment" that substance abuse is a problem by focusing, in the persuasion phase, on the further step of asking clients to make a *commitment* to pursue active treatment. In the persuasion phase, Community Connections uses "active user" groups that are confrontational and directive. Kofoed and his colleagues (1986) describe the use of "objective data" (such as breathalyzer or urine tests, psychiatric symptoms, and social or legal difficulties) to confront denial. Kofoed warns, however, that pushing clients into premature commitments may only result in additional, frustrating episodes of failure (Osher and Kofoed, 1989).

Assessment. The goal of assessment is to provide an understanding of both the mental disorder and the substance abuse problem (as well as the interactive effects) in order to fashion a comprehensive treatment approach. Lehmann, Myers, and Corty (1989) have emphasized that assessment is an ongoing process, geared to treatment phases. They emphasize that classification is a clinical tool, for making decisions about treatment alternatives at various stages of the client's treatment. At the initial assessment, it is important to clarify that both disorders are present and that one is not masking the existence of the other. In order to do so, both mental health and alcohol and drug assessment must be undertaken. For purposes of treatment matching, Minkoff (1989) has stressed distinguishing between secondary symptoms and primary disease, as well as attempting to establish the demarcation between substance abuse and dependence. In the Caulfield program, assessment begins during the acute stabilization phase, which may often include detoxification and abatement of symptoms associated with withdrawal. The Gladstone program emphasizes the importance of mental health and substance abuse personnel working together on assessments, involving much face-to-face contact and the opportunity to observe clients in nonclinical settings, such as in social clubs, at job sites, and in their homes.

Concomitant Treatment. Programs for persons with dual diagnoses have been developed under a variety of auspices. Regardless of auspice, however, these programs describe a phase of active treatment or rehabilitation, including a core set of mental health services and a core set of substance abuse treatment services. These services are provided either within the actual structure of the program or in direct relationship to the program. Table 3.1 outlines the core sets of services that may be provided directly by the program or by affiliation.

While the example programs discussed earlier vary in their focus and their capacity to provide these core services, they are all concerned with

Table 3.1. Core Elements of Mental Health and Substance Abuse Treatment Services

Mental Health Treatment Services	Substance Abuse Treatment Services
1. Crisis Management[a] Acute hospitalization Crisis residential alternatives	1. Detoxification[a] Medical Social
2. Stabilization Medication management	2. Pharmacologic treatments
3. Mental health interventions Individual, group, family therapy Day treatment Psychosocial rehabilitation	3. Recovery/rehabilitation interventions Alcohol and other drug education Group interventions Twelve-step groups (AA/NA)

4. Helping to establish positive social networks[a]
5. Providing residential opportunities[a] (alcohol- and drug-free housing)
6. Providing vocational opportunities[a]
7. Case management[a]
8. Family support and education[a]

[a] These services may be provided by the dual diagnosis program directly or be made available through other programs.

stabilizing psychiatric symptomatology and achieving and maintaining sobriety. In addition, they emphasize the development of new skills and new relationships to enable the person to remain sober. Though the type and sequencing of interventions are generally determined by individual need, most programs use some combination of individual counseling and group interventions that are peer-driven and abstinence oriented. Osher and Kofoed (1989) describe this as the development of a *culture of abstinence*. Gladstone emphasizes the need for acute treatment groups to be both confrontational and supportive, allowing the opportunity for clients to learn and practice new social and coping skills.

There are a few special issues that should be noted when programs begin the process of *hybridizing,* or combining these elements into a concomitant program or approach to treatment.

Mental Health Treatment. A particularly important aspect of dual diagnosis treatment is *medication management.* Beyond the problems of noncompliance with prescribed psychotropic medication are the possible negative interactive effects of alcohol and street drugs with psychotropic medication. Discussing these issues often leads to confusion over the "good drug/bad drug" issue. Clients may question why one drug is to be avoided while another is being prescribed. Clients must understand the role that psychotropic medications play in their rehabilitation.

Crisis management is critical if diversion from inappropriate service utilization is a goal. Crisis services within programs, such as in the Gladstone program, can be efficient and effective because staff will have access to information about the client's mental health and substance abuse histories, as well as current psychotropic prescriptions. As Safer (1987) and others have emphasized, substance abuse may exacerbate psychiatric symptoms and precipitate psychiatric hospitalization. Those programs managing crises (or providing triage for dually diagnosed persons in crisis situations) must be able to handle both psychiatric and substance abuse crises.

Social networks have been found to be an important reinforcer of alcohol and drug abuse behavior, especially among young adults with dual diagnoses (Lamb, 1982). Having opportunities to socialize, having access to positive recreational activities, and having a supportive peer group are stabilizing influences on clients who may otherwise drift from program to program or leave treatment altogether. Segal and Baumohl (1980) believe that the development of a social network for clients with disrupted natural social networks is so important that without it other conventional treatments will fail. Some programs, such as Community Connections and Gladstone, help clients to organize a peer network that will support their sobriety.

Substance Abuse Treatment. Regarding the substance abuse treatment elements, *alcohol and drug education* involves imparting simple information about the physiological and psychological effects of alcohol and drugs and, in the case of dually diagnosed persons, may also focus on the specialized effect these substances have on persons with brain disorders. Staff in some dual diagnosis programs report that they emphasize the connection of substance use with decompensation and rehospitalization, finding that many clients fail to make the connection on their own.

Group interventions are felt to be among the most powerful techniques to be used in substance abuse treatment and are included in most dual diagnosis programs. Long-term group support as well as assistance in confronting denial are seen as important. Programs vary somewhat in how confrontational versus supportive they are, and some groups are led primarily by professional staff while others are more peer-driven. The use of intensive confrontational tactics in group interventions remains somewhat controversial. While some mental health clinicians have seen confrontation as useful in promoting group cohesiveness, others warn that confronting more fragile psychotic clients may result in decompensation rather than insight. Again, individual assessment is critical to determining the appropriate use of any technique.

Referral to *Alcoholics Anonymous* (or *Narcotics Anonymous*) is very frequent in dual diagnosis programs because AA/NA meetings are accessible and available on a daily basis, unlike specialized dual diagnosis support groups. The opportunity of daily attendance at AA has offered many clients a better chance of maintaining sobriety (Kofoed, Kania, Walsh, and Atkinson, 1986). Concerns about AA usually focus on whether or not dual diagnosis clients "fit" in community Twelve-Step groups. In general, dually diagnosed persons require some preparation for AA. At the Caulfield Center, such preparation includes the assistance of recovering staff members in locating meetings suitable for dual diagnosis patients as well as education on how to make use of AA meetings (Minkoff, 1989).

Relapse Prevention/Aftercare. Many dual diagnosis programs encourage their clients to attend AA meetings and to participate in a sponsor relationship. For many substance abuse treatment programs, AA is the only kind of aftercare offered, due to funding or other constraints. In some programs, including Community Connections, an additional phase of treatment involves teaching clients about relapse, since lapses in sobriety are to be anticipated. Helping clients through early relapses is believed to be one way of preventing later ones, when clients may no longer be as connected to the treatment program (Osher and Kofoed, 1989).

Developing Linkages. Dual diagnosis programs usually must interact with two (mental health and substance abuse) or, in some cases, three (mental health, alcohol abuse, and drug abuse) systems of care. Some programs have been able to improve their programmatic efforts by addressing barriers to interagency and intersystem coordination, through the use of (1) cooperative agreements, (2) shared staffing, and (3) staff training.

Cooperative agreements are usually formal agreements between agencies or systems that set up key referral procedures and specify cooperative programming. In order for those agreements to be operational, and not just "paper" agreements, a spirit of collaboration and shared responsibility must be developed. Some programs invest significant administrative time in developing and maintaining these cooperative linkages, to facilitate system functioning.

Shared staffing refers to formal or informal agreements in which staff trained and employed in one system of care are assigned to programs in the other system to consult or to provide direct services. As mentioned previously, the Gladstone program employs a shared staffing arrangement. Shared staffing is one way to enrich the capability of programs without hiring new staff. To ensure flexibility in treatment approach, however, it is important that these shared staff have an understanding of both substance abuse and mental disorders.

Finally, *staff training* may be an effective mechanism for addressing philosophical and ideological barriers, as well as enhancing dual diagnosis treatment skills. Training may involve sharing information about mental and substance disorders, and sharing clinical experience in assessment, diagnosis, and treatment. Mental health program administrators in some areas have arranged for their staff to provide in-service training to the staff of the local substance abuse agency and vice versa. This has resulted not only in the transfer of useful information but also continued contact among the treatment personnel, promoting intersystem collaboration as well as expanding staff knowledge about dual disorders. One cautionary note is warranted. Considering the different backgrounds of the participants in cross-system training, simply putting people in the same room does not ensure that they will come to consensus. Mutual respect often follows from some period of working together, and may not be a reasonable expectation of training sessions.

Conclusion

This chapter has described four examples of hybrid, or integrated, dual diagnosis treatment programs as well as identifying the elements common to these programs: addressing phases of treatment, addressing engagement and motivation, providing for specialized assessment of both disorders and their interaction, providing simultaneous core treatment for both disorders, and developing support systems for relapse prevention. In addition, hybrid programs commonly develop techniques for addressing barriers to interagency and intersystem collaboration.

Because of the heterogeneity of the dual diagnosis population, all programs do not, and need not, look alike. Attending to the type and severity of psychiatric, as well as substance, disorder requires the specialization of programs. In addition, hybridization is not the only, nor is it necessarily the preferred, approach to delivering care to all persons with dual diagnoses. Possibly the reason that it has been the focus of much of the current program development for severely mentally ill persons is that there is so little historical evidence of success in attempts to provide parallel or coordinated treatment across service systems. That is not to say that such attempts are in vain. Some local service systems with a reasonable continuum of care in each sector have tried mechanisms such as intersystem case conferences to create, in effect, a working treatment team across system barriers. Others have proposed that case managers be used to cross system boundaries, accessing and coordinating care delivered by more traditional mental health and substance abuse treatment agencies (Willenbring, Ridgely, Stinchfield, and Rose, 1991).

Nevertheless, for those agencies, programs, and systems that wish to utilize a hybridized approach, the elements identified here will be useful in program development.

References

Alterman, A., Erdlen, D., and Murphy, E. "Effects of Illicit Drug Use in an Inpatient Psychiatric Population." *Addictive Disorders*, 1982, *7*, 231–242.

Bachrach, L. "The Context of Care for the Chronic Mental Patient with Substance Abuse." *Psychiatric Quarterly*, 1987, *58*, 3–14.

Bachrach, L., Talbott, J., and Meyerson, A. "The Chronic Psychiatric Patient as a 'Difficult Patient': A Conceptual Analysis." In A. Meyerson (ed.), *Barriers to Treating the Chronic Mentally Ill*. New Directions for Mental Health Services, no. 33. San Francisco: Jossey-Bass, 1987.

Cohen, M., and Klein, D. "Post-Hospital Adjustment of Psychiatrically-Hospitalized Drug Users." *Archives of General Psychiatry*, 1974, *31*, 221–227.

Galanter, M., Castaneda, R., and Ferman, J. "Substance Abuse Among General Psychiatric Patients: Place of Presentation, Diagnosis, and Treatment." *American Journal of Drug and Alcohol Abuse*, 1988, *14*, 211–235.

Hall, R., Popkin, M., and DeVaul, R. "The Effects of Unrecognized Drug Abuse on Diagnosis and Therapeutic Outcome." *American Journal of Drug and Alcohol Abuse*, 1977, *4*, 455–465.

Kofoed, L., Kania, J., Walsh, T., and Atkinson, R. "Outpatient Treatment of Patients with Substance Abuse and Coexisting Psychiatric Disorders." *American Journal of Psychiatry*, 1986, *143*, 867–872.

Lamb, R. "Young Adult Chronic Patients: The New Drifters." *Hospital and Community Psychiatry*, 1982, *333*, 465–468.

Lehmann, A., Myers, C., and Corty, E. "Assessment and Classification of Patients with Psychiatric and Substance Abuse Syndromes." *Hospital and Community Psychiatry*, 1989, *40*, 1019–1025.

McLellan, A., Luborsky, L., Woody, G., and others. "Predicting Response to Alcohol and Drug Abuse Treatments: Role of Psychiatric Severity." *Archives of General Psychiatry*, 1983, *40*, 620–625.

Minkoff, K. "Development of an Integrated Model for Treatment of Dual Diagnosis of Psychosis and Addiction." *Hospital and Community Psychiatry*, 1989, *40*, 1031–1036.

Osher, F., and Kofoed, L. "Treatment of Patients with Psychiatric and Psychoactive Substance Use Disorders." *Hospital and Community Psychiatry*, 1989, *40*, 1025–1030.

Ridgely, M. S., Goldman, H. H., and Talbott, J. A. *Chronic Mentally Ill Young Adults with Substance Abuse Problems: A Review of the Literature and Creation of a Research Agenda.* Baltimore: Mental Health Policy Studies, University of Maryland School of Medicine, 1986.

Ridgely, M. S., Goldman, H. H., and Willenbring, M. "Barriers to the Care of Persons with Dual Diagnoses: Organizational and Financing Issues." *Schizophrenia Bulletin,* 1990, *16,* 123–132.

Ridgely, M. S., Osher, F. C., and Talbott, J. A. *Chronic Mentally Ill Young Adults with Substance Abuse Problems: Treatment and Training Issues.* Baltimore: Mental Health Policy Studies, University of Maryland School of Medicine, 1987.

Safer, D. "Substance Abuse by Young Adult Chronic Patients." *Hospital and Community Psychiatry,* 1987, *38,* 511–514.

Segal, S., and Baumohl, J. "Engaging the Disengaged: Proposals on Madness and Vagrancy." *Social Work,* 1980, *25,* 358–365.

Stein, L., and Test, M. A. "Community Treatment of the Young Adult Patient." In B. Pepper and H. Ryglewicz (eds.), *The Young Adult Chronic Patient.* New Directions for Mental Health Services, no. 14. San Francisco: Jossey-Bass, 1982.

Willenbring, M., Ridgely, M. S., Stinchfield, R., and Rose, M. *Application of Case Management in Alcohol and Drug Dependence: Matching Techniques and Populations.* Rockville, Md.: National Institute on Alcohol Abuse and Alcoholism, 1991.

M. Susan Ridgely, M.S.W., is research associate in psychiatry and associate director of the Mental Health Policy Studies Program of the Department of Psychiatry, School of Medicine, University of Maryland.

Assessment of complex dual diagnosis patients requires a careful, systematic approach to evaluating diagnosis, severity, and motivation.

Assessment of Comorbid Psychiatric Illness and Substance Disorders

Lial Kofoed

While many patients suffer from both substance and psychiatric disorders, this comorbidity is often discovered only after much time, pain, and embarrassment. In this chapter I will review important dimensions of assessment for patients with comorbid disorders, specific assessment tools and techniques, challenges to the validity of assessment, and prognostic and treatment planning implications.

Overview

Appropriate diagnosis of comorbid disorders requires a realistic index of suspicion based on their frequency in *clinical* populations. Epidemiologic Catchment Area community data reveal that presence of a substance disorder increases the risk of psychiatric disorder (odds ratio 2.3 for alcoholism, 4.5 for drug use disorders); similarly, the risk of substance disorders is increased in persons with a psychiatric illness (odds ratio 2.7) (Regier and others, 1990). More important, these already high comorbidity rates *more than double* in persons seeking treatment. Comorbid psychiatric illness is found in 24 percent of alcoholics and 30 percent of drug addicts who have not sought treatment in the past year, but in 55 percent of alcoholics and 62 percent of drug addicts who have sought treatment. Unfortunately comorbidity is strongly associated with treatment noncompliance, treatment resistance, and chronicity of symptoms (Drake, Osher, and Wallach, 1989; LaPorte, McLellan, O'Brien, and Marshall, 1981; Lehmann, Myers, and Corty, 1989). Thus, it is necessary to consider comorbid illness in all patients, and to consider this possibility even more seriously when patients fail to respond to standard treatments for either psychiatric or substance disorders.

Assessment

Dimensions of assessment include diagnosis, severity of illness, and motivation for treatment. Few studies specifically examine implications of assessment for prognosis and treatment planning in dual diagnosis patients. Available studies focus on treatment of singly diagnosed populations or on treatment of single disorders. With regard to dual diagnosis patients, Lehmann, Myers, and Corty (1989, p. 1019) observed that "assessment and classification may be most usefully viewed as open-ended clinical procedures for planning treatment on a case-by-case basis." The open-ended nature of assessment, with diagnoses considered tentative in the face of changing data, cannot be overemphasized in the dual diagnosis patient. These complications must be borne in mind throughout this discussion of the dimensions of assessment.

Diagnosis

Diagnosis of Comorbid Substance Disorders. Assessment to establish the diagnosis of a substance disorder is the most useful first step in assessing dual diagnosis patients, for three reasons. First, the diagnosis can be reliably made early in assessment. Second, missing the diagnosis has serious implications, since unrecognized substance abuse will compromise psychiatric diagnosis and further assessment. Third, the implications of a positive diagnosis for treatment planning, especially given the need to focus on attaining sobriety, are valid regardless of other comorbidity.

Employing substance disorder assessment tools in addition to standard clinical interviews can be effective in overcoming the denial that characterizes these disorders. Denial can be understood as the inability of patients to admit the extent of their drug or alcohol use and to connect their use with its negative consequences. Such denial is clinically apparent even in severely ill dual diagnosis patients (Kofoed and Keys, 1988). Helzer and Pryzbeck (1988) found that although dually disordered alcoholic patients are more likely to seek medical treatment than uncomplicated alcoholics, they are no more likely to discuss their drinking with the treating physician. Similarly, Test, Wallisch, Allness, and Ripp (1989) found that schizophrenic patients were less likely to report frequent drinking or to consider heavy drinking problematic than their case managers.

Turning now to assessment tools for alcoholism, the CAGE (Mayfield, McCleod, and Hall, 1974) is a four-item questionnaire validated for use as a screening tool in nonpsychiatric populations. Drake and others (1990) examined the CAGE in schizophrenic patients. They found the CAGE to be 73.7 percent sensitive to both current and lifetime diagnosis of alcoholism using a cutoff score $\geq$ 2, with specificity for current alcoholism of 73.2 percent and lifetime alcoholism of 97.3 percent. Thus the CAGE is a useful screening instrument in dual diagnosis populations.

The Michigan Alcoholism Screening Test (MAST) (Selzer, 1971) has also been examined in dual diagnosis populations. It has been shown to have greater than 80 percent sensitivity but variable specificity (from 36 to 89 percent) in psychiatric patients (Hedlund and Vieweg, 1984). In a small study, Toland and Moss (1989) did not find the MAST useful in differentiating alcoholic and nonalcoholic schizophrenic patients, though alcoholic patients had greater mean MAST scores. The instrument generated false positives due to patient confusion of alcohol-related versus schizophrenic symptoms, and by its inability (inherent in the questionnaire design) to distinguish current from past problems. Drake and others (1990) found the MAST 84.2 percent sensitive for current and 86.8 percent sensitive for lifetime alcoholism in schizophrenic patients using a cutoff score of $\geq$ 5. Specificity for lifetime alcoholism was 81.1 percent, but specificity for current alcohol problems was only 57.1 percent. This again reflects the failure of the MAST to distinguish current from past problems.

A modification of the MAST, the Veterans Alcoholism Screening Test (VAST) (Magruder-Habib, Harris, and Fraker, 1982), imposes a time structure on the MAST questions, and in primary alcoholic populations is more sensitive and specific than the MAST. The VAST has not been studied yet in dual diagnosis populations.

Drake and others (1990) also examined sensitivity and specificity of a research interview using DSM-III-R criteria for assessing alcohol use disorders. In schizophrenics they found that the purposeful interview was 100 percent specific but only 73.7 percent sensitive to current alcoholism. This interesting finding suggests that the purposeful interview for an alcohol abuse diagnosis may miss a quarter of patients with such a diagnosis even in experienced hands. In addition, there may be difficulties with the DSM-III-R criteria for alcohol use disorders as applied to dual diagnosis patients; some data suggest that patients with severe psychiatric illnesses suffer adverse effects from surprisingly low levels of alcohol consumption (Drake, Osher, and Wallach, 1989).

Collateral informants are often helpful in determining the presence of substance disorders. Instruments such as the MAST or the VAST can be filled out by family members regarding the patient, with results that are sensitive and specific (Magruder-Habib, Harris, and Fraker, 1982). Similarly, Drake and others (1990) found that case manager ratings, incorporating longitudinal observations and collateral reports, were more sensitive and specific than research interviews.

Because of the diversity of other abusable drugs, it has not been possible to develop assessment instruments as succinct as those available for alcoholism. One of the more widely used structured interviews is the Addiction Severity Index (ASI) (McLellan, Luborsky, Woody, and O'Brien, 1980), which guides the interviewer through a series of questions about drug use and its consequences. This interview has been shown to effectively assess substance abuse problems when compared to other accepted measures; its sensitivity in comorbid populations is not known. However, the ASI does not provide specific diagnoses.

In younger patient populations, diagnosis of an alcohol problem should always raise the question of abuse of other drugs as well; conversely, few patients abuse other drugs without also experiencing periods of alcohol abuse.

The laboratory may be helpful in assessing substance disorders. Toxicologic study is a useful screening technique, but it is limited in several ways. First, drug use cannot automatically be equated with abuse (though this equation is more nearly true in dual diagnosis patients than in any other population). Second, given their inevitable inaccuracy, single positive reports must be used cautiously. Third, given the varying duration of detectability of various drugs and the often sporadic nature of substance abuse, toxicologic screening may lead clinicians to a false sense of security.

Diagnosis of Comorbid Psychiatric Disorders. The presence of substance abuse greatly increases the difficulty of establishing a psychiatric diagnosis, primarily because symptoms secondary to intoxication or withdrawal can mimic most psychiatric syndromes, especially during cross-sectional or time-limited observation (Penick and others, 1988). While prolonged deferral of psychiatric diagnosis and treatment until extended sobriety is achieved is often recommended, clinicians working with highly symptomatic dual diagnosis patients often have neither the means to enforce immediate sobriety nor the opportunity for lengthy observation in controlled settings. Delay may also be counterproductive for reasons discussed later. In addition, because most patients who *enter* substance abuse treatment with severe psychiatric symptoms remain more symptomatic than other patients throughout and after treatment (McLellan and others, 1983), evidence of significant psychiatric comorbidity soon after detoxification is likely to be clinically significant.

Studies of depressive symptoms in alcoholic patients using a variety of scales show reductions in symptoms with increasing duration of sobriety (Mayfield, 1985; Nakamura, Overall, Hollister, and Radcliffe, 1983; Willenbring, 1986). However, such scales are not precisely equivalent to DSM-III-R syndromatic diagnoses of major affective disorders, and cannot answer the question of *diagnostic* validity (Willenbring, 1986).

Affective symptoms that clear quickly with sobriety reflect symptoms secondary to substance abuse, and depression-focused psychotherapy or antidepressant medications are not appropriate. However, a substantial subgroup do suffer from a primary depressive disorder, which is less likely to remit spontaneously without specific treatment. Penick and others (1988) found that 21.2 percent of a cohort of alcoholic men remained depressed according to a psychiatric diagnostic interview a year after entering substance abuse treatment. Thus, it appears necessary to devise a way of distinguishing early in treatment between temporary depressive symptoms, which do not require specific treatment, and more chronic and significant symptoms. This would avoid delaying appropriate treatment for patients with clinically significant depression.

Willenbring (1986) compared the Hamilton Depression Scale (Ham-D) (Hamilton, 1960), the Beck Depression Inventory (BDI) (Beck and others, 1961), and the Depression Scale of the MMPI to diagnosis from a DSM-III guided clinical interview in alcoholics entering treatment. He found that the Ham-D showed the strongest correlation with the DSM-III diagnosis, and suggested that the BDI and MMPI are not useful screening scales. He also found, however, that Ham-D scores tended to show substantial improvement when repeated at twenty-one days, suggesting low specificity of identification of clinically relevant major depressive disorders.

Penick and others (1988) found somewhat greater symptom stability using the Psychiatric Diagnostic Interview, a DSM-III–compatible modification of Feighner and others' (1972) diagnostic interview. They found that at one-year follow-up, 52.7 percent of alcoholic subjects initially diagnosed as depressed still met diagnostic criteria for depressive disorder.

In assessing depressive symptoms in patients with substance abuse and schizophrenia (or other serious psychiatric illness), matters become profoundly complicated. There are no clear data to guide decision making in these multiply comorbid patients. Although either the DSM-III-R interview or the Ham-D may accurately identify major depressive disorder, the specificity of diagnosis in early sobriety using these instruments in primary alcoholics is poor, and specificity in comorbid populations even less certain.

Psychiatric disorders may be diagnosed in early sobriety (one to two weeks) using standard DSM-III-R criteria, and appropriate treatment can be initiated. However, the assessment process must remain open ended, because the diagnoses may change over time. Data on the stability of psychiatric syndromes diagnosed early in the course of alcohol treatment is provided by Penick and others (1988). Using a structured interview incorporating Feighner and others' (1972) and DSM-III criteria for fifteen common psychiatric illnesses, Penick and colleagues derived index diagnoses during initial hospitalization for alcohol treatment. They repeated the interview a year later, and compared diagnostic findings. Of the common codiagnoses, depression was positive at some time in 30.7 percent of subjects, and in 16.1 percent (over half of all depressed subjects) at both interview periods. Mania was present at some time in 10 percent, and in 3 percent at both times. Schizophrenia was present in 2.1 percent at some time, and in 0.4 percent at both times. Overall, excluding alcoholism, 55 percent of all subjects ever positive for a given diagnosis were positive at both time periods. About two-thirds of the discordance resulted from apparent symptom remissions; symptoms did not meet the diagnostic threshold at the follow-up interview. The other one-third of discordance was accounted for by new or worsened symptoms exceeding diagnostic threshold at follow-up but not at baseline. The authors note that in discordant cases the difference was usually one of degree rather than category. Most subjects reported similar symptoms at both time intervals, with discordance accounted for by varying symptom severity rather than differing symptom types. A large percentage of subjects in this study also had diagnoses of drug abuse, suggesting that additional substance abuse diagnoses did not invalidate psychiatric diagnosis. Overall, their data suggest that major psychiatric syndrome diagnoses are fairly stable even when diagnosed shortly after alcohol treatment begins. However, there is a significant rate of remission over a year of follow-up, so that clinicians need to recall the open-ended nature of the assessment process in this difficult population, and all initial psychiatric diagnoses and treatments need to be periodically re-evaluated.

Sequence and Diagnosis. There has been considerable discussion about the importance of time of onset of illness in the assessment of comorbidity. The reasoning behind this discussion seems sound. If substance abuse began first, then subsequent psychiatric symptoms may be secondary, and treatment of the substance disorder will eliminate the psychiatric comorbidity. The converse argument is also apparently sound. If substance abuse seems to be an attempt at "self-medication" of a specific psychiatric illness, then adequate treatment of the psychiatric symptoms may produce sobriety. Despite the logic in such reasoning, there is little evidence that such distinctions are valid, however. In patients with possible psychiatric illness predating substance abuse, several factors complicate the assumption that psychiatric treatment is sufficient for both disorders. The first is the difficulty of obtaining a valid history of symptom sequence, especially in the face of denial, which leads patients to delayed recognition of the onset of substance disorders. The second is the failure of the literature to demonstrate consistent diagnosis/drug of choice combinations, as would be expected if self-medication was a major cause of comorbid substance abuse (Lehmann, Myers, and Corty, 1989). In fact, some of the clearest relationships, such as that between stimulants and schizophrenia, are counterintuitive in terms of the self-medication hypothesis. Most patients abuse multiple classes of drugs.

Finally, the nature of abusable drugs (they reinforce their own use over time) and the delay between onset and recognition of abusive use suggest that by the time of diagnosis a "secondary" substance disorder may have assumed a life of its own. Patients learn to count on substance use to relieve aspects of their dysphoria in uniquely individual ways, and the self-reinforcing nature of abusable drugs leads to a conditioned expectation of relief that remains even when relief no longer occurs. Some individuals carry a genetic vulnerability that leads to substance disorders with relatively less exposure, but probably no one is immune from risk. Thus, substance abuse, even if initially secondary, eventually becomes self-sustaining and usually requires specific treatment at the point of diagnosis. The issue of secondary substance disorders remains of scientific interest, but is not currently of much help in clinical decision making.

Similar problems affect diagnosis of secondary psychiatric symptoms. Careful physical and mental status examination and toxicologic screening are required to minimize such errors as mistaking amphetamine intoxication or delirium tremens for schizophrenia. Toxicological screening, though not helpful for diagnosing withdrawal syndromes, probably should be incorporated into psychiatric ward admission protocols. Careful cognitive examination may prevent confusing delirium with functional thought disorder, avoiding inappropriate treatment. Objective data such as tachycardia and hypertension, evidence of tremor and hyperreflexia, and horizontal or vertical nystagmus can help diagnose an intoxicated or withdrawal state (Osher and Kofoed, 1989). Psychotic symptoms secondary to acute intoxication or withdrawal may require brief treatment with antipsychotic medication, but usually remit spontaneously within two weeks (Schuckit, 1984). However, prolonged abuse of some classes of drugs produces lasting psychological symptoms (McLellan, Woody, and O'Brien, 1979). For example, long-term stimulant abuse produces a symptom pattern characterized by progressive elevation of the MMPI hysteria, paranoia, schizophrenia, and mania scales, while long-term barbiturate abuse leads to progressive elevation of the MMPI depression scale as well as increased frequency of suicide attempts. Effects of long-term marijuana use may mimic the negative symptoms of schizophrenia. Distinguishing such symptoms from primary psychiatric illness is difficult, and requires careful ongoing assessment while maintaining abstinence. The development of treatment plans in such difficult situations is discussed later.

Severity. Symptom severity is an important element of assessment, and is generally best evaluated by clinical history and interview. Assessment scales may also be helpful. For example, severity of alcoholism can be reflected by MAST or VAST scores; severity of depression by Ham-D scores; and severity of other aspects of psychiatric illness by MMPI scale scores, SCL-90 scores, and so on. The ASI provides global ratings of severity in multiple problem areas, including alcohol and drug problem severity and psychiatric symptom severity. The psychiatric symptom severity rating from this instrument has been shown to predict poor treatment outcome in primary substance abuse treatment programs, making it potentially useful in evaluating dual diagnosis treatment programs.

Motivation. Assessment of motivation is an important aid to treatment planning. However, such assessment should not be used to exclude patients from treatment. Motivation is a *state*, not a trait, and may be modified by a variety of interventions (Kofoed and Keys, 1988; Osher and Kofoed, 1989). Motivation does appear to predict early sobriety in dual diagnosis patients; Ries and Ellingson (1990) have shown that self-assessments of motivation for sobriety on a five-point scale were associated with maintenance of sobriety a month after hospital discharge. This simple assessment technique thus appears quite valid and useful.

Assessment of motivation should include assessment for the presence of potentially coercive influences that may contribute to motivation. For mentally ill patients, coercion for treatment within the mental health system may take the form of threatened loss of housing or day programming due to substance-related behavior. Conversely, inducements for sobriety may include promised referral to improved housing or to vocational rehabilitation.

Similarly, legal issues may also influence motivation. Several studies have suggested that legal coercion (probation, deferred prosecution, or treatment as a sentence) is either neutral or associated with improved treatment retention compared to noncoerced patients in primary substance abuse treatment (reviewed in Shore and Kofoed, 1984). Limited data suggest that this is also true of dual diagnosis patients (Kofoed, Kania, Walsh, and Atkinson, 1986).

Implications of Assessment for Treatment Planning and Prognosis

Diagnosis

Substance Disorders: Type of Substance. Certain patterns of drug usage have specific treatment implications. A diagnosis of opioid use disorder suggests consideration of methadone maintenance or opiate antagonists such as naltrexone (Trexan); diagnosis of alcohol use disorder implies potential usefulness of disulfiram (Antabuse). However, most patients— and virtually all younger patients—are found to engage in patterns of polydrug abuse. Ries and Ellingson (1990) found that only two of seventeen dual diagnosis patients used alcohol alone. Thus, diagnosis of type of substances abused is less useful than was true in the past, as patients move from one drug class to another in seemingly random ways, related more to fashion and availability than pharmacology.

Psychiatric Disorders. Because most addiction treatment programs screen to exclude patients with severe psychiatric illness, there are few studies of the effects of specific diagnoses on substance abuse treatment outcome, and even fewer in programs specifically designed for dual diagnosis. The data that do exist are only valid in treatment approaches similar to those studied; there are likely to be specific interactions between diagnosis and type of treatment that are poorly understood.

In a small descriptive study, Kofoed, Kania, Walsh, and Atkinson (1986) found that non-character-disordered dual diagnosis patients in specialized outpatient treatment had treatment retention rates similar to uncomplicated substance abusing patients treated in nonspecialized programs. This study included no unipolar depressed patients. Ries and Ellingson (1990), in a small descriptive study of patients in inpatient dual diagnosis treatment, found the highest substance abuse relapse at one-month follow-up in bipolar patients, intermediate relapse rates in schizophrenic patients, and lowest relapse rates in depressed patients.

Diagnostic Interactions. There are suggestions of diagnostic interactions with potential prognostic significance. These include evidence of a preferential association of schizophrenia with stimulant use disorders, and consequent worse psychiatric and occupational outcomes than either nonabusing schizophrenic or nonschizophrenic stimulant abusing patients (McLellan, Woody, and O'Brien, 1979; Perkins, Simpson, and Tsuang, 1986; Schneier and Siris, 1987). Other interactions probably exist; their treatment implications are unknown. Further study of these interactions is very important.

Severity

Severity of Substance Abuse. Severity of substance disorders has not been strongly predictive of substance abuse treatment outcome (McLellan and others, 1983). Data suggest that the distinction between abuse and dependence as embodied in DSM-III had little prognostic significance (Schuckit, 1984) beyond suggesting a need for detoxification; consequently in DSM-III-R the "dependence" category was considerably broadened, and now includes many patients formerly diagnosed with only "abuse." Implications of the new DSM-III-R categories for the treatment requirements of dual diagnosis patients have yet to be studied.

For patients with serious psychiatric disorders, substance use appears to have negative consequences even at low use levels (Drake, Osher, and Wallach, 1989). Thus, boundaries between "use" and "abuse" are further blurred. If negative consequences of use can be documented and abstinence cannot be maintained, it is appropriate to recommend specific treatment for substance abuse.

Psychiatric Symptom Severity. A series of studies have demonstrated that increased severity of psychiatric symptoms at intake is associated with worse outcome across a variety of substance abuse treatment modalities, in both inpatient and outpatient settings (McLellan and others, 1983; McLellan, 1986). McLellan and colleagues (1983, 1986) found psychiatric symptom severity to be more predictive of treatment outcome than medical, legal, social, and substance abuse severity factors measured by the ASI (McLellan, Luborsky, Woody, and O'Brien, 1980; McLellan and others, 1983). These findings seem particularly robust because they were demonstrated in a sample of patients already screened for substance abuse treatment, with severe psychiatric illness excluded. Thus, even fairly moderate psychiatric symptoms are associated with worse treatment outcomes in a variety of substance abuse–focused treatment modalities.

The negative prognostic implications of symptom severity may not apply to programs that offer integrated mental health and substance abuse treatment, however. Four open clinical trials with dually diagnosed patients (one of schizophrenic patients, two of mixed groups of patients with major mental illnesses, and one of patients with post-traumatic stress disorder) have found that interventions aimed at reducing both psychiatric symptomatology and substance abuse produce treatment outcomes similar to those achieved in effective programs for primary substance abusers (Hellerstein and Meehan, 1987; Kofoed, Kania, Walsh, and Atkinson, 1986; Kuhne, Nohner, and Barage, 1986; Ries and Ellingson, 1990).

The relationship between psychiatric symptom severity and poor substance abuse treatment outcome does *not* depend on the cause of the symptoms; untreated organic affective disorder or organic delusional disorder secondary to substance abuse will complicate substance abuse treatment as surely as primary psychiatric illness. It appears that the clinical side of this complex issue can be resolved fairly simply. In patients with severe psychiatric symptoms that last beyond intoxication or the expected acute withdrawal period, successful substance abuse treatment will depend on reduction of psychiatric symptoms by appropriate treatment. The major value of assessment of psychiatric symptom severity is in treatment planning. Patients with high symptom severity require specialized programming to be treated effectively (Kofoed, Kania, Walsh, and Atkinson, 1986; Osher and Kofoed, 1989).

Motivation

Assessment of motivation allows placement of dual diagnosis patients in an appropriate treatment phase (Osher and Kofoed, 1989). When patients are poorly motivated for sobriety, initial efforts should focus on engaging the patient to accept the need for sobriety and for substance abuse and mental health treatment (Kofoed and Keys, 1988). In patients who are already strongly motivated, immediate entry into abstinence-oriented treatment and psychiatric rehabilitation is appropriate.

Motivation can be reassessed throughout treatment by attending to compliance. Laboratory testing is useful in ascertaining compliance with psychopharmacologic therapies, particularly lithium and tricyclic antidepressants. Such testing is also helpful in the differential diagnosis of inadequate treatment response. Similarly, toxicologic screening is useful for ascertaining continued abstinence.

Assessment as Treatment

The process of assessment also incorporates the initial steps of treatment: forming a therapeutic relationship, bringing problems into the open, discussing treatment options, and setting treatment limits, all within a context of ongoing respect and acceptance. If this can be done well, the assessment process sets the stage for a positive and productive treatment process.

There is growing understanding that persuading patients to accept treatment is an important and legitimate part of substance abuse treatment, with evidence in dual diagnosis patients (Kofoed and Keys, 1988) demonstrating that persuasive efforts can have a positive effect on treatment acceptance. Presenting the results of the assessment to the patient, with careful description of the symptoms, natural history, and likely course of both disorders, as well as treatment options and their probable effectiveness, is as appropriate for dual diagnosis patients as for patients with any medical diagnosis. Such matter-of-fact presentation is the foundation of the persuasive process, and can have a powerful impact in helping patients become free of their own guilt and shame about substance abuse or mental illness by modeling a nonjudgmental approach (Atkinson, 1985).

Conclusion

I have reviewed available studies and provided assessment guidelines based on available data for treatment planning. There are severe limitations in both our concepts and our instruments, and many instruments will have to be revalidated in specific dual diagnosis populations. Much more research about the etiologic interactions of specific substance disorders and specific psychiatric disorders is needed. Finally, available data provide only the broadest hints about the interactions of various diagnoses and treatments. I hope those of us treating these challenging and rewarding patients can renew our commitment to clinical science, continuing to generate and test clinical hypotheses rather than reaching premature conclusions about assessment and treatment issues. With continuing exploration, this complex field will avoid lockstep treatment approaches and continue to develop innovative and effective methods of treatment delivery for dual diagnosis patients.

References

Atkinson, R. M. "Persuading Alcoholic Patients to Seek Treatment." *Comprehensive Therapy*, 1985, *11*, 16-24.

Beck, A. T., Ward, C. H., Mendelson, M., Mock, J., and Erbaugh, J. "An Inventory for Measuring Depression." *Archives of General Psychiatry*, 1961, *4*, 561-571.

Drake, R. E., Osher, F. C., Noordsy, D. L., Hurlbut, S. C., Teague, G. B., and Beaudett, M. S. "Diagnosis of Alcohol Use Disorders in Schizophrenia." *Schizophrenic Bulletin*, 1990, *16*, 57-67.

Drake, R. E., Osher, F. C., and Wallach, M. A. "Alcohol Use and Abuse in Schizophrenia: A Prospective Community Study." *Journal of Nervous and Mental Disease*, 1989, *177*, 408-414.

Feighner, J. P., Robins, E., Guze, S. B., Woodruff, R. A., Winokur, G., and Munoz, R. "Diagnostic Criteria for Use in Psychiatric Research." *Archives of General Psychiatry,* 1972, *26,* 57-64.

Hamilton, M. "A Rating Scale for Depression." *Journal of Neurology, Neurosurgery, and Psychiatry,* 1960, *23,* 56-62.

Hedlund, J. L., and Vieweg, B. W. "The Michigan Alcoholism Screening Test (MAST): A Comprehensive Review." *Journal of Operational Psychiatry,* 1984, *15,* 55-65.

Hellerstein, D. J., and Meehan, B. "Outpatient Group Therapy for Schizophrenic Substance Abusers." *American Journal of Psychiatry,* 1987, *144,* 1337-1339.

Helzer, J. E., and Pryzbeck, T. R. "The Co-Occurrence of Alcoholism with Other Psychiatric Disorders in the General Population and Its Impact on Treatment." *Journal of Studies on Alcohol,* 1988, *49,* 508-512.

Kofoed, L., Kania, J., Walsh, T., and Atkinson, R. M. "Outpatient Treatment of Patients with Substance Abuse and Coexisting Psychiatric Disorders." *American Journal of Psychiatry,* 1986, *143,* 867-872.

Kofoed, L., and Keys, A. "Using Group Therapy to Persuade Dual-Diagnosis Patients to Seek Treatment." *Hospital and Community Psychiatry,* 1988, *39,* 1209-1211.

Kuhne, A., Nohner, W., and Barage, E. "Efficacy of Chemical Dependency Treatment as a Function of Combat in Vietnam." *Journal of Substance Abuse Treatment,* 1986, *3,* 191-194.

LaPorte, D. J., McLellan, A. T., O'Brien, C. P., and Marshall, J. R. "Treatment Response in Psychiatrically Impaired Drug Abusers." *Comprehensive Psychiatry,* 1981, *22,* 411-419.

Lehmann, A. F., Myers, C. P., and Corty, E. "Assessment and Classification of Patients with Psychiatric and Substance Abuse Syndromes." *Hospital and Community Psychiatry,* 1989, *40,* 1019-1025.

McLellan, A. T. "Psychiatric Severity as a Predictor of Outcome from Substance Abuse Treatments." In R. E. Meyer (ed.), *Psychopathology and Addictive Disorders.* New York: Guilford Press, 1986.

McLellan, A. T., Luborsky, L., Woody, G. E., and O'Brien, C. P. "An Improved Diagnostic Evaluation Instrument for Substance Abuse Patients: The Addiction Severity Index." *Journal of Mental and Nervous Disease,* 1980, *168,* 26-33.

McLellan, A. T., Luborsky, L., Woody, G. E., O'Brien, C. P., and Druley, K. D. "Predicting Response to Alcohol and Drug Abuse Treatments: Role of Psychiatric Severity." *Archives of General Psychiatry,* 1983, *40,* 620-625.

McLellan, A. T., Woody, G. E., and O'Brien, C. P. "Development of Psychiatric Illness in Drug Abusers: Possible Role of Drug Preference." *New England Journal of Medicine,* 1979, *301,* 1310-1314.

Magruder-Habib, K., Harris, K. E., and Fraker, G. G. "Validation of the Veterans Alcoholism Screening Test." *Journal of Studies on Alcohol,* 1982, *43,* 910-926.

Mayfield, D. "Substance Abuse in the Affective Disorders." In A. I. Alterman (ed.), *Substance Abuse and Psychology.* New York: Plenum, 1985.

Mayfield, D., McCleod, G., and Hall, P. "The CAGE Questionnaire: Validation of a New Alcoholism Screening Instrument." *American Journal of Psychiatry,* 1974, *131,* 1121-1123.

Nakamura, M. M., Overall, J. E., Hollister, L. E., and Radcliffe, E. "Factors Affecting Outcome of Depressive Symptoms in Alcoholics." *Alcoholism Clinical and Experimental Research,* 1983, *7,* 188-193.

Osher, F. C., and Kofoed, L. L. "Treatment of Patients with Psychiatric and Psychoactive Substance Abuse Disorders." *Hospital and Community Psychiatry,* 1989, *40,* 1025-1030.

Penick, E. C., Powell, B. J., Liskow, B. I., Jackson, J. O., and Nickel, E. J. "The Stability of Coexisting Psychiatric Syndromes in Alcoholic Men After One Year." *Journal of Studies on Alcohol,* 1988, *49,* 395–404.

Perkins, K. A., Simpson, J. C., and Tsuang, M. T. "Ten-Year Follow-Up of Drug Abusers with Acute or Chronic Psychosis." *Hospital and Community Psychiatry,* 1986, *37,* 481–484.

Regier, D. A., Farmer, M. E., Rae, D. S., Locke, B. Z., Keith, S. J., Judd, L. L., and Goodwin, F. K. "Comorbidity of Mental Disorders with Alcohol and Other Drug Abuse: Results from the Epidemiologic Catchment Area (ECA) Study." *Journal of the American Medical Association,* 1990, *264,* 2511–2518.

Ries, R. K., and Ellingson, T. "A Pilot Assessment at One Month of Seventeen Dual Diagnosis Patients." *Hospital and Community Psychiatry,* 1990, *41,* 1230–1233.

Schneier, F. R., and Siris, S. G. "A Review of Psychoactive Substance Use and Abuse in Schizophrenia: Patterns of Drug Choice." *Journal of Nervous and Mental Disease,* 1987, *175,* 641–652.

Schuckit, M. A. *Drug and Alcohol Abuse: A Clinical Guide to Diagnosis and Treatment.* New York: Plenum, 1984.

Selzer, M. L. "The Michigan Alcoholism Screening Test: The Quest for a New Diagnostic Instrument." *American Journal of Psychiatry,* 1971, *127,* 89–94.

Shore, J. H., and Kofoed, L. "Community Intervention in the Treatment of Alcoholism." *Alcoholism: Clinical and Experimental Research,* 1984, *2,* 151–159.

Test, M. A., Wallisch, L. S., Allness, D. J., and Ripp, K. "Substance Use in Young Adults with Schizophrenic Disorders." *Schizophrenia Bulletin,* 1989, *15,* 465–476.

Toland, A. M., and Moss, H. B. "Identification of the Alcoholic Schizophrenic: Use of Clinical Laboratory Tests and the MAST." *Journal of Studies on Alcohol,* 1989, *50,* 49–53.

Willenbring, M. L. "Measurement of Depression in Alcoholics." *Journal of Studies on Alcohol,* 1986, *47,* 367–372.

Lial Kofoed, M.D., is associate professor of clinical psychiatry at Dartmouth Medical School and currently directs the PTSD Clinical Team at the White River Junction VA Medical Center in White River Junction, Vermont.

New Hampshire's specialized dual diagnosis services include
continuous treatment teams and substance abuse treatment groups
within each mental health center. These services are embedded in
an extensive system of care for the dually diagnosed.

New Hampshire's Specialized Services for the Dually Diagnosed

Robert E. Drake, Linda M. Antosca, Douglas L. Noordsy,
Stephen J. Bartels, Fred C. Osher

The New Hampshire Division of Mental Health and Developmental Services (DMHDS), in collaboration with the state's Office of Alcohol and Drug Abuse Prevention and the New Hampshire–Dartmouth Psychiatric Research Center, began in 1987 to establish an integrated treatment system for all residents who were dually diagnosed with chronic mental illness and substance disorder. An overview of the system, the training program, and the related research projects has been presented elsewhere (Drake, Teague, and Warren, 1990; Teague and Drake, 1991; Teague, Mercer-McFadden, and Drake, 1989). In this chapter, we will briefly review the program and describe in detail with clinical examples two of the program's core components—regional continuous treatment teams and specialized substance abuse treatment groups.

New Hampshire's Mental Health Service System

Since this program may represent the first attempt to integrate treatment for dually diagnosed people as a specialty service throughout an entire state, we will begin with a brief description of New Hampshire's mental health service system. New Hampshire is a northern New England state with rural and small urban areas and a population of approximately 1.2 million people. The state is divided into ten mental health service regions, each with a primary community mental health center (CMHC). The only public psychiatric hospital in the state contains 144 beds and is located in Concord, at the geographic center of the state. Smaller, regional psychiatric units are, in most areas, contained within general hospitals.

Mental health care in the ten regions and the state hospital is carefully coordinated by the New Hampshire DMHDS, which is linked through contracts for clinical services and research with the Dartmouth Medical School. State-funded mental health services focus on the chronically mentally ill and have been developed over several years in accordance with the National Institute of Mental Health guidelines for community support programs (Stroul, 1989). In this system, case managers with caseloads of approximately thirty to forty coordinate treatment plans, continuity of care, and access to a comprehensive array of services.

With increasing evidence in New Hampshire as elsewhere that some clients were difficult to engage in community programs, the state began to develop continuous treatment teams in 1987. Based generally on the Training in Community Living model developed in Dane County, Wisconsin (Test, 1991; Test and Stein, 1976), these teams were intended to provide active outreach and community-based services for the hard-to-reach client. Because a large majority of the clients in this target population were dually diagnosed, the Research Center developed plans to make the continuous treatment teams specialists in dual diagnosis and to include them in a larger plan to integrate services throughout the state for this population. Consequently, DMHDS applied for and received assistance from the Robert Wood Johnson Foundation under its Mental Health Services Development Program to establish "system integration and specialized services for people with chronic mental illness and substance abuse problems." New Hampshire will receive Foundation funds for three years and will maintain the dual diagnosis program thereafter with public resources.

The program has three primary components: (1) integrated services; (2) systemwide training; and (3) planning, development, and coordination at state and regional levels. Services are integrated with special staff and training to evaluate and treat dually diagnosed patients throughout the system. This includes developing individual service plans in conjunction with the client, the family, and other caregivers; coordinating treatment across outpatient, inpatient, and residential treatment settings; and serving as liaison to the substance abuse system, the criminal justice system, and others involved in the care of the dually diagnosed. The training program and system oversight occur at the state and regional levels by bringing together mental health and substance abuse personnel, families, and consumers. A program director within DMHDS convenes the interagency advisory board and training activities at the state level and facilitates the development of similar working groups at the regional level.

Continuous Treatment Teams

At the center of New Hampshire's program are continuous treatment teams (CTTs)—multidisciplinary units that provide direct, comprehensive, long-term services to dually diagnosed clients and their support systems. CTTs serve clients who (1) meet DSM-III-R criteria for coexisting substance disorder and severe mental illness and (2) are considered candidates for more intensive services because they are not well engaged in treatment and are at risk for recurrent hospitalization or homelessness.

New Hampshire's CTTs combine the principles of intensive case management from the Training in Community Living model (Test, 1991; Test and Stein, 1976) with emerging concepts of dual diagnosis treatment (Drake, Osher, and Wallach, in press; Minkoff, 1989; Osher and Kofoed, 1989). They integrate substance abuse treatment into an array of direct services that include case management, crisis intervention, housing, skills training, vocational rehabilitation, supportive psychotherapy, medication monitoring, and family psychoeducation. Rather than putting the burden of integrating systems and interventions on the client, CTTs ensure the continuity of mental health and substance abuse treatments across services and over time.

Team Approach. Three to six clinicians, including a half-time psychiatrist, a nurse, at least one addiction specialist, and at least one specialist in chronic mental illness, comprise each CTT. Most of the clinicians have master's degrees in related fields. The team shares responsibility for each client and serves as a fixed point of responsibility for a relatively small set of clients (for example, fifty clients for a team of five clinicians).

Services are generally provided through intensive outreach in the client's natural environment rather than in the clinic. Because the team shares responsibility for all clients, each day begins with a team meeting to review the entire caseload and to develop plans for clients who are unstable or in crisis. Frequent team meetings allow team members to plan and coordinate activities, as well as to support and supervise each other. A team leader coordinates schedules and activities, but treatment planning, case reviews, and supervision are done as a team.

Through shared responsibility, each clinician's areas of expertise can be brought to bear on a particular client. For example, for a particular client, one clinician may provide medication education, a second teaches vocational skills, a third leads a substance abuse treatment group, and a fourth meets with the family. Since team members learn rapidly from each other in this model, their roles are fluid and may shift from day to day. Thus, the nurse has primary responsibility for coordination with inpatient nursing staff and for client education regarding AIDS and other medical problems but also participates in the full range of outreach, substance abuse counseling, and other services. One advantage of asking each clinician to learn a broad range of interventions is that CTTs attract clinicians who are flexible and eager to learn new skills.

The team approach has numerous other advantages. Clinicians can easily cover for each other during vacations or illnesses. They share the stress of demanding clients and frequent crises. They work in pairs when appropriate. For example, two clinicians often address crises in which the client and his or her family or support system could benefit from services simultaneously. Clients rapidly learn that they can contact any team member rather than one individual and appreciate the opportunity for greater access. Difficult relationships between a particular clinician and a particular client can be mitigated by the flexibility to shift and share responsibility. In practice, about one-third of the clients continue to relate to several clinicians over time, while others develop a stronger relationship with one clinician but continue to receive some services from others.

Dual Diagnosis Expertise. The central focus of New Hampshire's continuous treatment teams is the integration of mental health and substance abuse treatments. CTT clinicians offer substance abuse counseling to individuals, lead dual diagnosis groups in the mental health center (described below), and reach out to educate families about substance abuse. They also link clients to the existing substance abuse treatment system and to the self-help system by screening meetings for appropriateness, preparing them for the experience, attending meetings with them, and discussing the experience with them afterward.

Individual CTT clinicians typically start out with a background in either mental health or substance abuse treatment, but they rapidly learn to think more broadly about the challenges of dual disorders. In part these changes occur because of regular workshops, readings on dual diagnosis, and monthly didactic meetings with all of the CTTs and the Research Center staff. They are also encouraged to attend AA, NA, CA, Al-Anon, and COA meetings, which offer a unique opportunity to learn about issues related to chemical dependency, to understand and appreciate the self-help system, and to confront one's own experiences with alcohol and other drugs. Most of their learning occurs, however, in the daily experience of struggling as an interdisciplinary staff with a recurrent set of problems.

Historical stereotypes about dual diagnosis—such as that mental health problems are always manifestations of chemical dependency or that substance abuse always occurs secondary to underlying psychiatric disorders— disappear rapidly as clinicians learn to appreciate the complexity of treating two chronic, relapsing disorders. Nuances of the clinical relationship become the focus of team meetings: for example, discussions of titrating support against reinforcing, or enabling, addiction and of tolerating versus confronting denial in the face of psychosis. Team members must be flexible and willing to take an empirical approach to complex clinical problems for which dogmatic approaches are often inadequate.

As the CTTs develop experience treating dual diagnosis, their influence spreads in concentric layers. They work directly with a small set of treatment-refractory clients; they lead dual diagnosis groups that are open to all CMHC clients; and they educate and consult with families, fellow clinicians, and other care providers (for instance, in hospitals, shelters, housing programs, and the criminal justice system). Perhaps most important, their successes begin to engender optimism and enthusiasm for treating dual diagnosis throughout the system.

Longitudinal Treatment. Integrated treatment is a process that takes place over years rather than weeks or months. The common problem of front-loading substance abuse treatment is overcome by the team's long-term commitment to provide continuity and to facilitate recovery over years. Heuristically, substance abuse treatment is expected to occur in four stages: engagement, persuasion, active treatment, and relapse prevention (Osher and Kofoed, 1989). These refer to developing a trusting relationship (engagement), helping the client to perceive and accept the problem of substance abuse (persuasion), achieving stable abstinence (active treatment), and maintaining abstinence (relapse prevention). In practice, progress is highly individual with lengthy periods of engagement and persuasion, frequent relapses to prior stages, and unexpected returns to controlled drinking by some patients. In a parallel process that is not always in synchrony, the client learns to manage his or her mental illness in similar stages: engagement, acknowledgment, self-management, and relapse prevention.

For clients who have histories of many failures and difficulty engaging in treatment, the CTT approach may be particularly effective. The emphasis on intensive outreach by a team allows for considerable help with practical matters and maximal flexibility in the engagement process. As described in the following case, legal leverage may facilitate engagement. Psychoeducational work with families may also be helpful. Once clients are engaged, the consistency and continuity of CTT supports them through other stages of substance abuse and mental health treatments.

Case Example. Jack was a thirty-year-old, homeless, single male with a long history of both schizophrenia and alcoholism. When Jack faced criminal charges for threatening behavior, his attorney was referred to the CTT for help. After meeting with Jack and his lawyer, the team recommended to the court six months of mandatory community treatment in lieu of incarceration. The judge accepted this recommendation and thereby paved the way for successful engagement. To engage Jack, who was extremely paranoid about the mental health system, team members met him regularly at a local coffee shop and used a loan fund to treat him to breakfast. Expectations were kept at a minimum while a relationship developed.

As the weather turned cold, Jack grew tired of living in his car and agreed to an admission in the local hospital's mental health unit. On discharge he was less paranoid and moved into an apartment that the CTT helped him to secure. He remained medication compliant but continued to abuse alcohol intermittently. When his probation was reviewed at the end of six months, Jack was released from court jurisdiction but continued his relationship with the CTT.

Soon thereafter Jack began working and, with a regular income, resumed his pattern of daily drinking. Team members continued to be supportive and also pointed out the consequences of his drinking: stopping medications, losing his rent money, inconsistent work behavior, and a renewal of angry outbursts. A breakthrough occurred when Jack discovered that his boss was an alcoholic in recovery. With the boss's encouragement, he agreed to a medical checkup and learned that he had gastritis and early liver damage. Consequently, he began attending the CTT's dual diagnosis group (the Alcohol Education Group) in the CMHC. The team as well as the group continued to make connections between Jack's drinking and the problems in his life, while exploring with him more adaptive ways to handle boredom and stress.

After countless invitations, Jack finally agreed to attend an AA meeting with one member of the team and several clients. He sat in the back row and was filled with delusions about the meeting. The team carefully processed the meeting afterward with Jack and the other clients. He learned that recovery is a slow and halting process, and struggled to reduce his alcohol intake.

When the team sensed that Jack was ready for detoxification, they prepared him for an inpatient program. Active treatment was underway. The CTT helped the inpatient alcohol treatment unit to modify their usual confrontational style and met daily with Jack on the unit. Nevertheless, after three days, Jack left the program, walked home feeling both relief and despair, and resumed his drinking. The team interpreted Jack's brief participation as a commendable effort and expressed their respect for his decision. His failure to obtain sobriety was understood as part of the recovery process. Jack was surprised at their continued positive regard.

At this point, each period of abstinence is seen as a success. The number of days that Jack drinks per month continues to decrease, while his work performance, medication compliance, and social behaviors improve. Though not linked to AA, he continues to attend the CTT's Alcohol Education Group. He is not yet completely abstinent, but abstinence is now his goal. After two years of CTT intervention, he is considerably more stable and expresses more hope for his future.

Substance Abuse Treatment Groups

Many dually diagnosed individuals have difficulty using traditional alcohol and drug treatment programs and self-help groups. We therefore provide substance abuse groups that are tailored specifically to their needs within the mental health center setting. Two types of substance abuse groups correspond to the persuasion and active treatment phases of treatment. Persuasion groups are designed for clients who have not yet acknowledged that substance use is a problem; they are psychoeducational, interactive, and supportive. Active treatment groups are for clients who are committed to working toward abstinence; they use behavioral principles of substance abuse treatment in a group format.

Persuasion Groups. These groups are intended to help clients perceive how substances complicate their lives. Although persuasion groups were developed by Kofoed and Keys (1988) for inpatient units, we have adapted the concept for outpatient settings. The term *persuasion* is a slight misnomer since these groups are primarily educational. The Alcohol Education Group is a typical name.

The groups have two leaders, one with expertise in treating chronic mental illness and the other with expertise in treating addictive disorders, and at least one is a member of the CTT. Groups are held weekly, often shortly after the weekend so that periods of heavy drug and alcohol use are likely to be fresh in clients' minds. Brief sessions reduce the intensity and enable clients with limited attention spans to attend. Some groups run for forty-five minutes, while others have two twenty- to thirty-minute sessions separated by a short break. Leaders meet during the break and after the group to review the process and to plan strategy.

Groups are open to all clients, but weekly attendance is encouraged. Since initial attendance is usually a problem, the groups serve refreshments, include activities, and are extremely supportive. Acknowledging a problem with alcohol or other drugs is not a prerequisite, and AA ideology is specifically avoided. Case managers encourage resistant clients to attend by including the group in treatment plans, providing transportation, and scheduling events important to the client (such as a weekly paycheck) close to the time of the group. They sometimes arrange compulsory attendance as a condition of state hospital discharge, probation, or parole.

Persuasion groups are not confrontational. They assume instead that genuine acknowledgment of a substance abuse problem occurs over time in the context of peer group support and education. The stated goal of the group is to help members learn more about the role that alcohol and other drugs play in their lives.

Group leaders provide some didactic material on alcohol, other drugs, and mental illness, but they expend most of their efforts facilitating peer interactions and feedback about substance use. They actively limit the level of affect, monitor psychotic behaviors, and maintain the group's focus on substance abuse. For example, since a member who becomes agitated or delusional while speaking can be stimulating and frightening to other group members, the leaders calmly interrupt the speaker, extract some thread of the original topic from the delusional material to translate for the rest of the group, and thank the speaker for his or her comments. Members are allowed to leave early if they need to. Those who are reluctant to participate are invited to contribute at least once or twice during each meeting.

Persuasion group sessions often begin with a review of each member's use of alcohol and other drugs over the previous week. This discussion must be nonjudgmental so that members feel safe in reporting their use honestly. As a member discusses a recent period of intoxication, the rest of the group helps to identify antecedents, including internal emotional states, and consequences of use. All members are encouraged to contribute to this process, perhaps offering advice or relating a similar experience. Relevant films, short readings, or group outings are occasionally used to stimulate interest and discussion, but lengthy didactic presentations are avoided because members rapidly lose interest. Leaders field questions and provide brief educational information on addiction, the effects of various substances on physical and mental health, the concept of denial, and the interactions between drugs and medications. Group members often ask leaders about their own use of alcohol and other drugs. Leaders are typically open about their use; those who are recovering from addiction may share their own experiences, while those who are not honestly relate their own choices and suggest that having a mental illness may increase one's sensitivity to the adverse effects of substance use.

Case Example. Bruce was twenty-four years old when he came to the CMHC for treatment following many years of unremitting psychosis. He was referred to the Alcohol Education Group when his case manager became aware of his regular marijuana and alcohol use. In the group Bruce reported his belief that he had damaged his brain with LSD in adolescence and caused himself to hear voices. He said that drugs were bad for his brain and regularly stated his intention to quit using marijuana, alcohol, and cigarettes, but he always reported using again by the next meeting. He stated that alcohol helped him to fall asleep, and that he used marijuana for religious purposes. His speech was often disorganized and tangential. He usually rocked in his seat during the group and often asked to leave early.

The group leaders helped Bruce to communicate more effectively by summarizing his comments for others. Group members explained to him that his marijuana and alcohol use were probably increasing the severity of his symptoms, counteracting the beneficial effects of his medication, and leading to the need for higher doses of the medication. Bruce discovered a familial component to his substance abuse by developing a genogram of addicted relatives on the chalkboard as part of a group exercise. Over two years he became more comfortable in the group and stayed longer, sometimes for an entire session. As he gradually discontinued using marijuana and moderated his alcohol use, group members gave him feedback on the beneficial effects.

Active Treatment Groups. These groups are focused, behavioral, and oriented toward abstinence. Members, who are working toward a common goal of abstinence, are more active and confrontational. Although not required, attending self-help meetings is actively encouraged as an adjunct to attaining sobriety, and the group work often focuses on developing the skills to negotiate a self-help program successfully.

Behavioral principles of addiction treatment (Monti, Abrams, Dadden, and Cooney, 1989) guide active treatment groups. This approach is less stimulating than some others and addresses the development of skills that dually diagnosed clients often lack. Members learn social skills through the group interaction and use one another for support and assistance in attending self-help meetings. They are trained in assertiveness, giving and receiving criticism, drink or drug refusal skills, and managing thoughts about alcohol or other drug use. They learn to use food, music, or exercise as substitutes for alcohol or drug use. They also learn imaging to get beyond cravings for substances and to change positive images of alcohol or drug effects into images of hangovers, withdrawal, psychotic symptom exacerbation, and other negative consequences of substance use.

Moreover, members learn to recognize situations that increase their risk of substance use, and to use relapse prevention techniques for managing these situations. For example, relaxation training and principles of sleep hygiene are used to regain control over anxiety and insomnia that may lead to the use of alcohol or other drugs. Many members need help with concrete situations, such as learning how to set limits on substance abusing friends. Members are encouraged to write down their internal or interpersonal struggles during the week so that they can work on them in the group. Leaders help them to label and manage emotional experiences that they had been obliterating with substance use and to appreciate the gradual improvements in their mental health and stability that come with sobriety. Members often gain a greater sense of responsibility for managing both of their illnesses during this process.

Case Example. April came to recognize that her regular marijuana use increased her paranoia and auditory hallucinations after two years in a persuasion group. She decided to stop smoking marijuana following a hospitalization for an exacerbation of psychotic symptoms because she never wanted to return to the hospital again. Early withdrawal had taken place in the hospital, but she used the active treatment group (termed the Second Step Group) to discuss her cravings for marijuana and to develop skills for resisting the impulse to return to smoking marijuana again. Other members related similar experiences during their first six months of abstinence, supported her decision to quit, and pointed out that she would have to go through withdrawal all over if she smoked again.

April attended a few NA meetings at the encouragement of the group leaders, but was too anxious to continue. She discovered in the active treatment group that her concern about her boyfriend's drinking also increased her craving for marijuana, and she learned to let go of her attempts to control his drinking. After two brief episodes of marijuana use led to immediate paranoia, she was able to sustain abstinence. Three months later, her psychiatrist reduced her neuroleptic dose because her psychotic symptoms were markedly diminished. She continues to attend the persuasion and active treatment groups regularly to support her abstinence.

Separate Versus Combined Groups. The persuasion and active treatment approaches can be provided within one group or in two separate, sequential groups. Even when separate groups are operating, there is considerable overlap in functions. When specialty dual diagnosis treatment groups are first started in a mental health center, one group may suffice until several members are prepared to move on to the active treatment phase. Separate groups permit the intensity and style of the group to be tailored to the specific members. On the other hand, separate groups may be too small (less than six members) and siphon off all of the currently abstinent members from the persuasion group. We encourage members who join the active treatment group to continue coming to the persuasion group as role models and to help move the group norm of the persuasion group in the direction of abstinence. Clients at this level can often benefit from the opportunity to attend groups more than once a week.

Conclusion

New Hampshire's dual diagnosis treatment system began only five years ago. The initial success of the program has led to refinements of the clinical interventions, continual updating of the training program, experimentation with new innovations such as various models of residential treatment, and several research projects. One clear and important effect is in the area of hope. Armed with training, skills, and enthusiasm, CTT clinicians are eager and confident in identifying and treating dual disorders individually and in groups. Their expertise and enthusiasm have rapidly infected the rest of the mental health system. In addition, the abilities of the mental health and substance abuse systems to collaborate have increased markedly. They are now linked at all levels through administrative contracts, clinical demonstrations, research grants, working relationships, and the experience of successfully treating shared patients.

References

Drake, R. E., Osher, F. C., and Wallach, M. A. "Homelessness and Dual Diagnosis." *American Psychologist,* in press.

Drake, R. E., Teague, G. B., and Warren, S. R. "New Hampshire's Program for People Dually Diagnosed with Severe Mental Illness and Substance Use Disorder." *Addiction and Recovery,* 1990, *10,* 35–39.

Kofoed, L. L., and Keys, A. "Using Group Therapy to Persuade Dual-Diagnosis Patients to Seek Substance Abuse Treatment." *Hospital and Community Psychiatry,* 1988, *39,* 1209–1211.

Minkoff, K. "An Integrated Treatment Model for Dual Diagnosis of Psychosis and Addiction." *Hospital and Community Psychiatry,* 1989, *40,* 1031–1036.

Monti, P. M., Abrams, D. B., Dadden, R. M., and Cooney, N. L. *Treating Alcohol Dependence: A Coping Skills Training Guide.* New York: Guilford Press, 1989.

Osher, F. C., and Kofoed, L. L. "Treatment of Patients with Psychiatric and Psychoactive Substance Abuse Disorders." *Hospital and Community Psychiatry,* 1989, *40,* 1025–1030.

Stroul, B. A. "Community Support Systems for Persons with Long-Term Mental Illness: A Conceptual Framework." *Psychosocial Rehabilitation Journal,* 1989, *12,* 9–26.

Teague, G. B., and Drake, R. E. "Mental Health Services Research Through a Public-Academic Liaison: A Comparison of Two Case Management Models." In *Proceedings of the First Annual Conference of the National Association of State Mental Health Program Directors Research Institute.* Arlington, Va.: National Association of State Mental Health Program Directors, 1991.

Teague, G. B., Mercer-McFadden, C., and Drake, R. E. "New Hampshire's Program for People with Dual Diagnoses." *TIE Lines,* 1989, *6,* 1–3.

Test, M. A. "The Training in Community Living Model: Delivering Treatment and Rehabilitation Through a CTT." In R. Liberman (ed.), *Handbook of Psychiatric Rehabilitation.* New York: Pergamon Press, 1991.

Test, M. A., and Stein, L. "Practical Guidelines for the Community Treatment of Markedly Impaired Patients." *Community Mental Health Journal,* 1976, *12,* 72–82.

Robert E. Drake, M.D., Ph.D., is director of the New Hampshire–Dartmouth Psychiatric Research Center.

Linda M. Antosca, M.S.W., is a case manager on the continuous treatment team of West Central Services in Lebanon, New Hampshire, and is a research associate with the New Hampshire–Dartmouth Psychiatric Research Center.

Douglas L. Noordsy, M.D., is the psychiatrist on the West Central Services continuous treatment team and a research associate with the New Hampshire–Dartmouth Psychiatric Research Center.

Stephen J. Bartels, M.D., is a clinical consultant to the state's dual diagnosis program. In addition, he is a research associate with the New Hampshire–Dartmouth Psychiatric Research Center.

Fred C. Osher, M.D., formerly directed New Hampshire's statewide dual diagnosis training program and is now with the Office of Homelessness at the National Institute of Mental Health.

The step-by-step approach to integrated treatment for multiple disorders described in this chapter can be replicated at minimal cost in any type of mental health treatment program or service.

An Integrated Treatment Approach for Severely Mentally Ill Individuals with Substance Disorders

Kathleen Sciacca

According to the Alcohol, Drug Abuse, and Mental Health Administration (ADAMHA) (Ridgely, Osher, and Talbott, 1987), at least 50 percent of the 1.5 to 2 million Americans with severe mental illness abuse illicit drugs or alcohol, compared to 15 percent of the general population. This finding is consistent with earlier epidemiological studies reporting that 25 to 50 percent of newly admitted psychiatric patients have concomitant drug and/or alcohol abuse problems (Simon, Epstein, and Reynolds, 1968; Crowley, Chesluk, Dilts, and Hart, 1974; Davis, 1984; Kofoed, Kania, Walsh, and Atkinson, 1986). Similarly, in New York State, the Commission on Quality of Care for the Mentally Disabled (1986) found that 50 percent of the patients admitted for psychiatric care had alcohol or drug abuse that required treatment. Despite this high prevalence of combined mental illness and substance abuse, treatment resources are scarce. This author's review (1989a) of 100 clients in psychiatric outpatient services in New York State who had received extensive psychiatric care and who were known substance abusers revealed that 61 of the clients had never received substance abuse treatment. The remaining clients received minimal attention to their substance abuse, and had never been in any form of sustained substance abuse treatment. Many of these clients accepted the lack of availability of substance abuse services, and kept their substance abuse problems to themselves. Clearly, in many patients, mental illness, drug addiction, and alcoholism are not encountered as discrete disorders. Yet those services that are available for these patients are divided by funding sources, admission criteria, treatment methods, and staff training and philosophy (Ridgely, Goldman, and Willenbring, 1990).

Rectifying the lack of treatment resources for multiply diagnosed patients requires a comprehensive approach, integrating mental health and addiction treatment in a single program design. Multiple disorders are often undiagnosed by professionals who specialize in serving distinct populations (Ridgely, Goldman, and Willenbring, 1990). Addiction professionals may believe that mental illness is a symptom or manifestation of substance abuse; mental health professionals may believe that substance abuse is a symptom of mental illness. Neither group is therefore likely to provide effective treatment for multiply diagnosed patients in their usual treatment setting.

The purpose of this chapter is to describe an integrated treatment model that the author has developed, and that has been applied successfully to the treatment of mental illness, chemical abuse, and addiction (MICAA) throughout New York State and in other states across the country. The first step in describing this model is to clarify diagnostic terminology. Next, we will identify the limitations of traditional substance abuse and mental health treatment approaches, followed by an in-depth discussion of the MICAA treatment model itself.

Diagnostic Terminology

Diagnostic clarity is the first step in planning successful treatment. To address the problem of multiple diagnoses of mental illness and substance abuse, clinicians from either addiction or psychiatric backgrounds must learn to make the diagnosis for each disorder using the clear diagnostic criteria outlined in the DSM-III-R (American Psychiatric Association, 1987). In addition, each service system must expand its resources to provide protocols for the assessment and diagnosis of the multiple disorders regularly encountered. Interactive effects of multiple disorders must be explored on an individual basis, and consideration of which disorder came first, while perhaps etiologically important, should not deter the diagnosis and treatment of persistent conditions that are evident simultaneously in the present.

The term *dual diagnosis* is ambiguous (for example, mental illness and mental retardation are dual diagnoses). The term *mentally ill chemical abusers* or MICA was introduced by the New York State Commission on Quality of Care for the Mentally Disabled (1986) and has since had an additional "A" added for *and Addicted*: hence, MICAA. The commission's report made it clear that the term denoted individuals with severe, persistent mental illness, accompanied by chemical abuse and/or addiction. The following list sums up the characteristics of MICAA:

1. Severe mental illness exists independently of substance abuse; persons would meet the diagnostic criteria of a major mental illness even if there were not a substance abuse problem present.

2. MICAA persons have a DSM-III-R, Axis I (American Psychiatric Association, 1987) diagnosis of a major psychiatric disorder, such as schizophrenia or major affective disorder.
3. MICAA persons usually require medication to control their psychiatric illness; if medication is stopped, specific symptoms are likely to emerge or worsen.
4. Substance abuse may exacerbate acute psychiatric symptoms, but these symptoms generally persist beyond the withdrawal of the precipitating substances.
5. MICAA persons, even when in remission, frequently display the residual effects of major psychiatric disorders (for example, schizophrenia), such as marked social isolation or withdrawal, blunted or inappropriate affect, and marked lack of initiative, interest, or energy. Evidence of these residual effects often differentiates MICAA from reputations of substance abusers who are not severely mentally ill.

To differentiate persons who have severe alcohol and/or drug addiction with associated symptoms of mental illness, but who are not severely mentally ill, the term *chemical abusing mentally ill* or CAMI has emerged. These persons can be described as follows:

1. CAMI patients have severe substance dependence (alcoholism; heroin, cocaine, amphetamine, or other addictions), and frequently have multiple substance abuse and/or polysubstance abuse or addiction.
2. CAMI persons usually require treatment in alcohol or drug treatment programs.
3. CAMI persons often have coexistent personality or character disorders (DSM-III-R, Axis II) (Solomon, 1982).
4. CAMI patients may appear in the mental health system due to "toxic" or "substance-induced" acute psychotic symptoms that resemble the acute symptoms of a major psychiatric disorder. In this instance, the acute symptoms are always precipitated by substance abuse, and the patient does not have a primary Axis I major psychiatric disorder.
5. CAMI patients' acute symptoms remit completely after a period of abstinence or detoxification. This period is usually a few days or weeks, but occasionally may require months.
6. CAMI patients do not exhibit the residual effects of a major mental illness when acute symptoms are in remission.

The program described in this chapter is designed specifically for MICAA patients, not for CAMI patients. This is not to say that CAMI patients do not present the same problems of diagnosis and treatment as do MICAA patients. In fact, CAMI patients may sometimes be more problematic because of the manipulative aspects of their coexisting character pathology. Nonetheless, once CAMI patients are identified, it is often best that they be referred back to the addiction treatment system. It may be detrimental and regressive for those addicts who are not severely mentally ill to get caught up in some aspects of the mental health system.

Traditional Treatment Approaches

Now, let us describe characteristics of "traditional" treatment within each system.

Traditional Addiction (Substance Dependence) Treatment Approaches. This treatment can be characterized as follows:

1. Criteria for admission to alcohol and drug treatment programs traditionally emphasize willingness and motivation. The person who is "seeking" services must be aware of the problems substance abuse has caused and must be "ready" and "motivated" to engage in treatment, agreeable to participating in the treatment process as outlined, willing to accept the consequences of faulty participation, and agreeable to abstinence from all substances. MICAA patients often cannot meet those admission criteria. In addition, many MICAA patients who are motivated are excluded because some programs do not admit persons who are taking prescribed medications.

2. Alcohol and drug *detoxification* programs, by nature, are exceptions. These programs accept active (often unmotivated) users, usually hospitalize them from three to seven days, and provide medication to alleviate withdrawal. Completion of detoxification is frequently a criterion for admission to other forms of treatment. Unfortunately, MICAA patients may also be specifically excluded from many traditional detoxification programs, due to the lack of adequate staffing or staff training.

3. Traditional programs for alcoholism and drug addiction treatment are often intense and highly confrontational. Clients are confronted by professionals and peers in an effort to break down denial regarding the adverse effects of substance abuse, and the degree of the severity of the addiction. Confrontation is also employed in individual and group sessions to address maladaptive behaviors and character pathology. Some program models conduct marathons as an additional means of breaking down defenses. But many experts denounce the use of confrontation with MICAA clients, deeming it antitherapeutic and unnecessary (Sciacca, 1987b).

4. Finally, traditional addiction treatment emphasizes the concept of "hitting bottom" as a necessary prerequisite to sobriety (that is, patients must experience severe losses or deterioration in order to perceive that they need help for addiction). For MICAA patients, however, "hitting bottom" can mean decompensation into severe psychosis and regression in all areas of functioning. This is *not* recommended. Sciacca (1987b) has advocated that MICAA clients be maintained at a stable level, and that progress in substance abuse treatment should proceed from that level.

Traditional Mental Health Treatment Approaches for the Severely Mentally Ill. These are the standard procedures for treating this group:

1. Criteria for admission to mental health programs emphasize that the client is suffering from a major mental illness. Clients who manifest overt substance disorders may be excluded from treatment on the assumption that the substance disorder is "primary." Many clients may therefore conceal their use of substances for fear of rejection from treatment (Sciacca, 1987b). Clients are generally *not* "seeking" treatment for substance abuse problems.

2. Mental health treatment programs accept clients who are unmotivated. Many clients are unmotivated to receive treatment for mental illness, but are cajoled into participating. For MICAA patients, denial and lack of motivation regarding substance abuse are quite common. Consequently, MICAA patients in denial of substance abuse are frequently admitted to traditional mental health programs, but then find there are no programs that address that denial, or that address substance abuse at all.

3. Mental health programs are supportive, not confrontational. Interventions focus on helping clients to maintain fragile defensive structures. Although this approach is helpful for mental illness, such programs are often so nonconfrontational that substance abuse is never addressed at all, and clients are effectively enabled to continue in a self-destructive course.

4. Mental health treatment programs are often not accepting of the problem of substance abuse. Clinicians not well trained in dealing with MICAA patients may be judgmental and critical, and fail to recognize alcoholism and drug addiction as physiological diseases. Clients may not feel comfortable discussing their substance abuse in such a setting, just as they are not likely to feel accepted discussing their mental illness in traditional substance abuse programs.

The MICAA Treatment Program: Overview

In the MICAA treatment model first developed by Sciacca in 1984 (Sciacca, 1987b), programming is based on the nonjudgmental acceptance of all symptoms and experiences related to *both* mental illness and substance abuse. Patients are engaged in supportive peer groups that encourage candid discussion of all illness-related experiences to foster group identification and cohesion.

MICAA treatment groups are implemented as a component of existing mental health treatment, or as a part of an integrated program exclusively for MICAA. MICAA groups have been developed in a wide range of treatment programs, including short- and long-term inpatient hospitals, admission units, community residences, shelters, day treatment programs, continuing care programs, case management services, and outpatient clinics (Sciacca, 1987a).

The format is as follows. Selected patients receive mental health treatment as usual, and attend MICAA groups once or twice per week in lieu of other program activities. Group sessions last from forty-five to ninety minutes; the recommended group size is eight. In more acute inpatient settings, groups may meet more frequently and focus on shorter-term goals (such as stabilization of acute symptoms and setting up ongoing substance abuse services after discharge; and assisting clients to recognize substance abuse as a possible precipitating factor in their psychosis).

The MICAA treatment process begins by engaging the client to relate to the area of substance abuse, using interventions that *precede* traditional substance abuse treatment readiness. Interventions include a nonconfrontational approach to denial (Sciacca, 1987b) that assists clients through the process of attaining traditional readiness by emphasizing engagement through education rather than confrontation and consequences. For clients in high denial, imposing consequences for substance use is not only irrelevant, it may serve to disengage clients from treatment altogether. Before beginning MICAA treatment, however, rules regarding substance abuse should be established by the mental health program to ensure a safe environment. Unsafe or potentially disruptive conditions, such as behavior that is aggressive, violent, or dangerous to self or others, whether or not due to intoxication, cannot be tolerated in any component of the client's treatment. Similarly, selling drugs is a criminal offense and also cannot be tolerated. Further, actively intoxicated clients are not included in MICAA groups or other areas of treatment and may be referred for crisis intervention, detoxification, or psychiatric hospitalization. Once procedures to address such crises are in place, and safety is assured, a more leisurely process of engagement can occur.

Let us consider the MICAA treatment process by looking at a client in extreme denial, who denies substance use and is averse to participating in substance abuse services. The MICAA group leader provides the following sequential approach.

Phase I: Client in Denial

Step 1: Initial Contact Occurs. In any treatment setting, clients may be identified for referral to a MICAA group program either during the intake process or during ongoing treatment. In either case, the primary clinician or case manager informs the client that there is a special program, and that an appointment can be set up for the client to meet with the leader of that program to learn more about it. If the client is willing, contact with the MICAA group leader is arranged, either formally or informally. The MICAA group leader, once in contact with the client, conducts the pregroup interview to engage the client and prepare him or her for attending the MICAA program. Note that the primary clinician does *not* prepare the client for MICAA group attendance; this is done only by the trained group leader.

If the client refuses the initial contact with the MICAA group leader, the referring/primary clinician is advised to continue to educate and engage the client through statements of concern, such as, "I am concerned that if you were to drink alcohol with your medication you may become too rapidly intoxicated." Statements of concern that relate directly to the client's own experience may eventually gain credence, and may assist the client to get beyond the extremely resistive state. This approach may proceed as long as necessary (at times, for many months) to engage the client in agreeing to make the initial contact with the MICAA program.

Step 2: The Pregroup Interview Is Held. The MICAA leader begins the pregroup interview by informing the client that there is a special program that addresses both mental health symptoms and the use of alcohol and drugs, and that such a service has been useful to many clients in the mental health system. The client may respond with outright denial of his or her need for such a program, giving reasons such as "I don't use substances" or "I have no problem with substance abuse." The MICAA leader may respond in a nonthreatening way by stating, "There were indications in your history that you might have a problem with substance use, but if you don't agree that's okay. Meanwhile, why don't I tell you about this program to see if there is any aspect of it that may be of value to you, or any contribution you may be able to make to the program." Maintaining an atmosphere of collaboration is an essential strategy throughout the interview. The immediate objective is to sustain the interview long enough to explain the four components of the MICAA group process.

The *first* component is the *supportive* nature of the group process. Clients in denial are asked, "Even though you don't see substance abuse as a problem for yourself, do you think you could be supportive of the other group members who are seeking help for their substance abuse?" The MICAA group leader accepts the denial state, while at the same time setting the tone for a supportive group process. Most clients respond affirmatively to the question, and their ability to contribute is inherent in that response. Clients are informed that abstinence is not required, and that they will encounter various stages of readiness in other group members: "In our group there are persons like yourself who don't think they have a substance abuse problem; there are also persons who think they may have a problem but are not sure they want to stop using; there are persons who believe they have a problem and want to abstain, but are not yet able to do so; and there are persons who know they have a problem and who are successfully abstaining." This information prepares clients to accept the varying readiness levels in others, and helps to eliminate discussion regarding comparisons with other clients.

The *second* component is the *educational* aspect of the process. The MICAA leader attempts to establish a reason for the person in denial to participate by asking, "In this group we learn a lot about alcohol and drugs.

Do you have any interest in learning about this?" Clients who have denied any involvement with substances may at this point in the interview—when it is clear that we are not going to break down their denial—comfortably express interest in receiving education. Interest in education is an acceptable purpose for the client's participation, and is clearly acknowledged as such by the MICAA group leader.

Specific education on both mental illness and substance abuse is an essential part of the treatment process. Areas covered include: mixing medication with substances; the symptoms and syndromes specific to each disorder; the forms of treatment utilized for each disorder; the physiological disease concepts for each disorder in contrast to moral judgment and stigma; and the process of rehabilitation and recovery for each disorder, in contrast to chronic hopelessness and despair.

The *third* aspect of the interview informs the client that *outside speakers* (such as members of AA and NA, physicians, case managers, and so on) are invited to discuss various topics. Some clients find it attractive that the self-help group speakers will be invited to speak to them in the mental health setting, particularly if they have been resistant to, yet curious about, Twelve-Step programs. This part of the interview sets the tone for an open group process that includes others besides the leaders and the group members.

The *fourth* component of the process is the creation of an atmosphere of *receptivity to learning*. Clients are asked if they believe they will be able to view the educational materials and the experiences of others in an open-minded way, and to consider that they may learn something new in the process.

The pregroup interview is regarded as the beginning of the treatment process. At the completion of the interview, clients will be engaged to attend the group or not. If not, a time will be set up to meet with the client again, and an offer to allow the client to attend one session may be made. For clients who are not comfortable in groups, the leader may also offer to assist the client in adjusting by setting up additional individual meetings.

For those clients who do agree to attend, the pregroup interview is designed to establish a purpose for each client's participation (such as helping others, interest in education, hearing speakers, and so on). For the client in denial, this tends to eliminate the client's experience of "not knowing" what he or she is doing in a substance abuse program.

The interview is also designed to identify positive aspects of the person's eventual participation. All experiences the client may convey regarding his or her knowledge of substance abuse are highlighted by the leader as potential contributions: "Since you say you once lived with someone who was a substance abuser, sharing your experience with others may be very helpful to them."

In summary, the pregroup interview serves as a valuable tool to shape the group process into one that is meaningful and therapeutic, by encouraging peer support, growth and change, and sharing of knowledge and experiences in a nonthreatening environment, before the client even enters the group. It also serves as a guide for the leader to assess aspects of the process with which clients may have difficulty. Clients who make nonsupportive statements, for example, are taught how to participate more appropriately, and may even be re-interviewed in order to be helped to identify more effective responses to use while attending groups.

Step 3: The Client Begins to Attend the MICAA Group. In the early stages of group participation, when clients are still in high denial, educational materials are provided regarding numerous aspects of alcohol abuse, drug abuse, and mental illness. The objective is to get clients simply to "talk about" alcohol and drugs. During this early phase of the process, the use of written materials, guest speakers, videos, and films allows clients to participate in discussions of important topic areas in an impersonal, nonthreatening way. Educational materials are presented in a way that is specifically designed to elicit the opinions and knowledge of group members. For example, rather than directly teaching clients that marijuana may cause panic attacks, the MICAA leader asks clients what *they* think about such statements in the educational materials presented; then clients in denial may safely talk about "others they know" who have had a marijuana-induced panic attack. Such discussion usually results in the group validating or coming to the consensus that the information is accurate; the leader then concretizes the fact that a consensus has been reached. This process fosters the integration of didactic information with personal experience, and encourages a learning experience that is internalized rather than memorized.

Step 4: Group Discussion of Substance Abuse Is Fostered. The client is now talking generally about alcohol and drugs in the group setting. The most important focus during this phase is building necessary trust to assure clients that it is safe for them to begin to discuss their own use of substances openly in the group. Trust is developed by the leader through conveying a realistic understanding of substance abuse, substance dependence, and the recovery process, and through taking every opportunity to dispel the "moral" model of the willful substance abuser who is bad and socially deviant. Educational materials and information address adverse effects of substance abuse, as well as treatment available. Through encouraging open discussion, the leader learns how each individual perceives substance abuse, and provides positive reinforcement when clients talk about their own use. Thus, candid statements about continuing use are commended, and leaders indicate that the value of the group process depends on discussion of what is really happening for people, not what they think others would like to hear. AA and NA speakers are asked to tell their stories when they are invited to speak to the groups, thus further providing the group with a model of self-disclosure without shame or denial. MICAA clients may identify with an AA speaker in one session, and then go back to denying substance use in the next session. The object, however, is not to catch clients in lies, or corner them into admissions. Rather, the process of denial is allowed to unfold at a pace that is comfortable for the client. Consequently, clients remain at this level for weeks or several months before moving on to phase II.

Phase II: The Unfolding of Denial

Step 5: The Client Begins to Talk About His or Her Own Use of Substances. Talking about one's own use is not synonymous with experiencing substance abuse as problematic. Clients may initially discuss the positive experiences they have had when using substances, such as euphoria, relaxation, or symptom reduction. The leader does not argue directly with a client's subjective positive experience, but instead, gently explores the possibility that adverse experiences may be present as well by inquiring about how the client felt as the substance was wearing off, and whether symptoms of mental illness were exacerbated at any point. The leader may also inquire about the specific effects of various substances, for example by asking a cocaine abuser if he or she lacked energy or felt depressed in "coming down" off the drug. In addition, such inquiries provide the leader with information on the client's specific patterns of use and reasons for continuing to use. Common reasons for use include "self-medicating" psychotic symptoms, alleviating boredom, anxiety, or depression, and facilitating socialization. Other members of the group are encouraged to share their own positive and negative experiences with using substances for these reasons.

Once the client can admit—in the group—to *using* substances (though not necessarily to *abusing* substances), a thorough assessment is performed by the leader in a private interview. This assessment provides more information about the client's current substance use and substance use history, which in turn can be used by the leader to facilitate further openness in the group process.

Step 6: The Client Recognizes That Substance Abuse Is a Problem (Though He or She May Still Be Actively Using Substances). If we recall that our starting point was the person who denied any use of substances at all, we can see that important progress has been made. Each increment of participation, understanding, learning, and insight is a necessary part of the process. Progress is based on these factors and on the reduction of denial, *not* on the reduction of substance use or abstinence, unless that has occurred.

At this point the client usually has identified the adverse effects of one substance that disrupts his or her life the most. Through candid discussion and more open reporting of the negative consequences, the client can receive increasing feedback from other group members and the leader that helps him or her to recognize that this substance use is problematic. Once this occurs, the client can be engaged in further discussion—in the group—of how he or she plans to address the problem.

Step 7: The Client Becomes Motivated to Abstain. The client's decision to share a wish to become abstinent is based on the existence of a trusting alliance with the leader and other group members who are enlisted to assist with this goal.

The client usually begins to approach abstinence by trying to cut down on or eliminate the use of the most disruptive substance he or she is using. Exploration takes place in the group regarding patterns of use of that particular drug, the possibility of physical addiction and/or need for detoxification, the skills and strengths that the client needs to employ to attain abstinence, the triggers that may evoke use of the substance, and other areas in which the client needs to change in order to attain abstinence. The client is assisted to recognize the necessary treatment interventions and supports that will promote abstinence, and is now amenable to receiving specific recommendations and suggestions from the leader and the group. In a sense, the client is now *in treatment* for the first time, and is strongly commended for acknowledging his or her substance abuse problem, expressing motivation to change, and having the willingness to accept help. These are labeled as strengths and positive attributes.

Phase III: Movement Toward Abstinence
In this phase, the client's level of readiness to work on abstinence is at the level required by traditional substance abuse programs. However, the client may not be at this level of readiness for all substances abused.

Step 8: Active Treatment to Promote Abstinence Is Employed. In the group, interventions such as contracting for abstinence are employed. A client may be asked to go one day without the substance and report back to the group. Clients who have had the "illusion of control" may now realize for the first time that they are not in control of the use of the substance, due to the difficulty or inability they experienced in carrying out the contract. This may be frightening, but by now the MICAA group has become a secure, supportive environment for the denial to break down safely. Clients may now begin to realize the need for additional support to gain control of the substance use, and may begin to attend AA, NA, or other supportive adjunctive programs. As they gain control over the substance, the group explores the skills and strengths they are employing in doing so. In the event of a relapse, the group will help the client to call on these strengths, skills, and strategies in order to regain control.

Once some stability is attained, rehabilitation and recovery begin. The client is helped to recognize the positive effects of abstinence, such as more positive self-esteem, fewer crises, reduction of adverse effects, more energy, improved relationships, and so on. Clients begin to learn how to cope with issues in their lives without the use of substances, and to develop new techniques for dealing with feelings and promoting socialization.

Relapses and relapse prevention, including early recognition of relapse signs, are important topics for education during this later phase; educational materials from earlier phases can be repeated very effectively at this time.

Note that most clients abuse more than one substance. However, a client's success at gaining control over the most disruptive substance may not readily translate into the recognition that all substances are problematic. The recognition of addiction to one substance may lead clients to consider that they are addicted to other substances (including nicotine and caffeine), but further work in the group is necessary, exploring the adverse effects of each substance, before a commitment to attempt total abstinence will occur.

Step 9: Total Abstinence Is the Goal. Total abstinence from all substances is the goal of treatment for all MICAA clients, and working toward this goal proceeds for as long as necessary (often for years). Time-limited programs must therefore make provisions for continuity of the MICAA process after the program is completed.

In order to maintain abstinence, clients are taught to utilize available adjunctive support networks. Traditional Twelve-Step recovery programs (AA, NA, CA) are recommended but not required. Interested clients are helped to utilize these programs in ways that are most comfortable and useful for them as individuals. This process takes place within MICAA groups, where clients who attend Twelve-Step programs discuss both successful and unsuccessful experiences. In addition to attending recovery programs, clients work on developing other substance-free social networks and activities; participation in social clubs, community activities, and additional therapy is encouraged.

MICAA Support Programs

Self-led, self-help support programs specifically for MICAA clients are very effective adjuncts to more generic support programs in helping MICAA clients maintain abstinence. Such groups have begun to emerge in scattered locations throughout the country, both within the traditional AA network ("Double Trouble" meetings) and within the traditional mental health system.

"Helpful People in Touch," a Consumer Program for MICAA. Sciacca (1990) has developed a specific format for developing an MICAA support program, and for training recovering MICAA patients to become peer group leaders. This program, called "Helpful People in Touch," has attracted and engaged MICAA consumers who are not amenable to participating in traditional mental health or addiction treatment models.

In this program, the role of the peer group leader includes structuring participation of all members in discussions and decision making, and ensuring completion of group tasks such as shopping for refreshments, preparing coffee, collecting dues, taking minutes, and so on. Near the close of each meeting, the members decide the format and content of the next meeting. This may include selecting reading materials, films, or videos; choosing a topic for discussion; or simply deciding to have an open discussion.

Meetings take place in the evenings, usually once every other week, and last for about ninety minutes. Meetings are monitored, but not led, by a professional who remains on the premises and is available to assist participants with requests for materials, or to handle difficult situations such as attendance by intoxicated individuals.

MICAA-NON, a Program for Families and Friends of MICAA. Families and friends of MICAA clients are vital supports who suffer along with these clients, yet very often lack knowledge and understanding regarding multiple disorders. Traditional AMI programs are extremely helpful regarding mental illness, but frequently do not address the complexity of living with MICAA patients. Alanon programs are sometimes helpful, but often fail to address the severity and complexity of patients with coexisting mental illness.

In order to provide these families with a support program specific to their needs, the MICAA-NON program (Sciacca, 1989b) has been developed to help families help themselves by focusing on their own needs, rather than being totally involved with the needs of their MICAA relatives.

Families of MICAA clients frequently deny or hide their relative's substance abuse due to feelings of guilt or shame. In MICAA-NON meetings, families learn that just as they did not cause their relative's mental illness, they also did not cause his or her substance disorder. As a result, they can more openly discuss their painful experiences, as well as advocate more effectively for improved and more comprehensive services.

A great deal of education and outreach is necessary to initially (and continually) bring MICAA families together. MICAA-NON groups are led by professionals. Groups are usually started by agencies who have MICAA treatment programs, and led by staff from these programs. Participation is never limited to families of MICAA persons affiliated with the agency; once a group has begun, it is open to all families in the community. The local AMI chapters are notified of such meetings, and families who attend MICAA-NON but are not AMI members are encouraged to join that support network as well. MICAA-NON groups are held in the evenings, usually every other week or once a month. Meetings last for about ninety minutes, and content usually includes education and support. MICAA-NON leaders find that their work with MICAA clients is greatly enhanced by their acquired understanding of family issues, while participating families become better able to understand and help their MICAA relatives through increased empathy and detachment.

Implementing MICAA Treatment and MICAA Support Programs

The integrated MICAA group treatment program just described, along with the ancillary support programs ("Helpful People in Touch" and MICAA-NON) can be readily implemented in traditional mental health programs, as a component of existing services, through the following process.

Administrative Support. Obtaining clear, unqualified administrative support is an essential first step in implementing MICAA groups in a treatment program. Program leadership can demonstrate such support to staff by distributing information about the planned MICAA groups with an accompanying message of unequivocal commitment to the MICAA program.

Screening. MICAA clients presently in attendance at the program are identified either by existing knowledge of their substance use, or by the administration of a brief screening instrument. (The author uses a modified CAGE questionnaire; see Mayfield, McCleod, and Hall, 1974.) All clients admitted into the treatment program are administered the CAGE questionnaire at intake to ensure that all potential MICAA referrals are identified, and to determine the number of individuals requiring MICAA services and the number of groups and group leaders required.

Staff Development. First, *sensitization of all staff and clients (MICAA or not) about the diseases of alcoholism and drug addiction* is done prior to the development of specific MICAA programming. This ensures broad familiarity with the basic concepts of MICAA treatment and helps the staff and clients as a whole to understand and accept the new program. Second, *recruitment of program staff as MICAA group leaders* begins by identifying those staff who express a strong interest in providing MICAA services. Finally, *group leader education* takes place as an in-service process (if most of the staff work for a single institution) or as an interagency group (where staff members from numerous agencies are participating). As mental health professionals, the group leaders are not expected to be substance abuse experts, but rather substance abuse "liaisons." As a "liaison," a group leader may comfortably tell a client that he or she does not know the answer to a particular question, and provide the answer at a later time. Liaisons are taught to use an exploratory approach when providing MICAA treatment, and to feel comfortable joining in the group learning process.

Education proceeds by building on the knowledge and skills inherent in the liaison's ability to treat mental illness. The disease and recovery concepts of alcoholism and drug addiction parallel those of mental illness. Four essential parallels that guide treatment are: (1) Each disorder has active symptoms. (2) In each disorder, symptoms can be brought into remission. (3) In each disorder, bringing symptoms into remission is not a cure, because each illness is a potentially relapsing disease. (4) Treatment focuses on bringing symptoms into remission, and then developing strategies for preventing relapse.

Having realistic expectations regarding change and recovery reduces staff burnout and frustration. Moral and judgmental beliefs about substance abuse are dispelled, and liaisons are taught to dispel these beliefs in others.

Education content includes (but is not limited to) information about substance disorders, individual substances, available substance abuse treatment programs, interactive effects of multiple disorders, interactions of prescribed medications with illicit substances, and principles of providing MICAA treatment individually and in groups.

Liaisons are specifically taught the skills necessary to provide the treatment process outlined in this chapter. This entails: conducting pregroup interviews, administering assessments, developing treatment plans for multiple disorders, developing group leadership skills, providing appropriate interventions at each stage of the process, collaborating with adjunct services such as drug/alcohol detoxification programs, collaborating with other mental health professionals who may be serving group members, reporting/recording progress relevant to the group process and individual progress, and so on. Some liaisons learn to conduct MICAA-NON groups; others learn to monitor "Helpful People in Touch" consumer self-help groups.

As part of their participation in MICAA group leadership meetings, liaison staff review pertinent literature and provide educational materials to their co-workers. In effect, liaison staff become substance abuse resources to the team or agency they work with.

Conclusion

The MICAA treatment programs described in this chapter have been implemented within numerous service settings across the country, and have been demonstrated to be successful and cost effective, generally requiring no more than four hours per week of staff time devoted to MICAA services and education (Sciacca, 1987a). Many MICAA clients who have attended these programs have attained long-term abstinence (more than one, two, or three years), and others have been maintained in the community at a functional level that far surpasses their previous frequent recidivism due to increased control of their substance abuse. Agencies that implement these programs quickly become more comprehensive in their provision of services for multiply disordered clients, and do not have to search fruitlessly for solutions to the "MICAA problem."

Clearly, controlled research further testing the usefulness of this program model is needed. The author is currently in the process of developing a research study to accomplish this goal.

References

American Psychiatric Association. *Diagnostic and Statistical Manual of Mental Disorders.* (3rd ed.) Washington, D.C.: American Psychiatric Association, 1987.

Crowley, T. J., Chesluk, D., Dilts, S., and Hart, R. "Drug and Alcohol Abuse Among Psychiatric Admissions." *Archives of General Psychiatry,* 1974, *30,* 13-20.

Davis, D. I. "Differences in the Use of Substances of Abuse by Psychiatric Patients Compared with Medical and Surgical Patients." *Journal of Nervous and Mental Disease,* 1984, *172,* (11), 644-647.

Kofoed, L., Kania, J., Walsh, T., and Atkinson, R. "Outpatient Treatment of Patients with Substance Abuse and Coexisting Psychiatric Disorders." *American Journal of Psychiatry,* 1986, *143* (7), 867-872.

Mayfield, D., McCleod, G., and Hall, P. "The CAGE Questionnaire: Validation of a New Alcoholism Screening Instrument." *American Journal of Psychiatry,* 1974, *131* (10), 1121-1123.

New York State Commission on Quality of Care for the Mentally Disabled. *The Multiple Dilemmas of the Multiply Disabled: An Approach to Improving Services for the Mentally Ill Chemical Abuser.* Albany: New York State Commission on Quality of Care for the Mentally Disabled, 1986.

Ridgely, M. S., Goldman, H. H., and Willenbring, M. "Barriers to the Care of Persons with Dual Diagnoses: Organizational and Financing Issues." *Schizophrenia Bulletin,* 1990, *16* (1), 123-132.

Sciacca, K. "Alcohol/Substance Abuse Programs at New York State Psychiatric Centers Develop and Expand." *This Month in Mental Health* (New York State Office of Mental Health), 1987a, *10* (2), 6.

Sciacca, K. "New Initiatives in the Treatment of the Chronic Patient with Alcohol Substance Use Problems." *TIE Lines,* 1987b, *4* (3), 5-6.

Sciacca, K. "Mental Illness, Alcoholism, Substance Abuse, Multiple Disabilities . . . Whose Patient? Whose Treatment Approach?" Paper presented at the annual meeting of the American Orthopsychiatric Association, New York, Apr. 1989a.

Sciacca, K. "MICAA-NON, Working with Families, Friends, and Advocates of Mentally Ill Chemical Abusers and Addicted (MICAA)." *TIE Lines,* 1989b, *6* (3), 6-7.

Sciacca, K. "Introduction to Program Development for Comprehensive Services for Mental Illness, Chemical Abuse, and Addiction (MICAA)." Paper presented at the 34th annual conference of the American Association for Partial Hospitalization, Philadelphia, Aug. 1990.

Simon, A., Epstein, L. J., and Reynolds, L. "Alcoholism in the Geriatric Mentally Ill." *Geriatrics,* 1968, *23* (10), 125-131.

Solomon, J. "Alcoholism and Affective Disorders." In J. Solomon (ed.), *Alcoholism and Clinical Psychiatry.* New York: Plenum, 1982.

Kathleen Sciacca, M.A., is the founding executive director of Sciacca Comprehensive Service Development for Mental Illness, Drug Addiction, and Alcoholism (MIDAA) in New York City and is a mental health program specialist for the New York State Office of Mental Health. She is a nationally known consultant, program developer, lecturer, and seminar leader.

Most integrated treatment programs originate in the mental health system; this chapter describes a dual diagnosis program that originates in the addiction system as a modification of a traditional therapeutic community.

Modifying the Therapeutic Community for the Mentally Ill Substance Abuser

Peggy McLaughlin, Bert Pepper

Homelessness of marginal populations has become a problem in our cities nationwide. Although there are many precipitants to homelessness, the most intractable sector of the homeless population seems to be those who are both mentally ill and addicted to drugs or alcohol. Other chapters in this book describe innovative programs for the dually diagnosed homeless that are based in the mental health system. In this chapter we will describe an integrated treatment model that originated in the substance abuse system, as a modification of a traditional therapeutic community for substance abusers.

The Therapeutic Community

The term *therapeutic community (T.C.)* came into use in Great Britain prior to World War II; it was used to describe the new movement to unlock mental hospital wards and involve psychiatric patients in a social recovery unit based on the cooperative efforts of patients and staff.

In the 1950s Maxwell Jones and other British pioneers introduced the concept of the psychiatric hospital T.C. in the United States, but the term fell into psychiatric disuse during the 1960s. However, in that same decade it found a new form and a new home in the treatment of drug addicts.

In the 1960s psychiatrists and others who were pioneering in the treatment of heroin addiction developed residential programs for addicted persons and used the name T.C. There are now drug abuse T.C.'s in many parts of the United States. The transition has been so complete—from mental health to substance abuse—that many people are unaware that the term originally belonged to the psychiatric hospital (Campbell, 1989).

The drug abuse T.C., as it is commonly constituted, consists of a highly structured social rehabilitation residential program with a desired length of stay of one and a half to two years. Usually the addicted person is accepted into an orientation phase that lasts approximately one month. During this time stringent behavioral modification reward-and-punishment measures are used to orient the new resident. For example, during orientation there are no visitors and the resident is not allowed to leave the facility. All privileges must be earned by active positive behaviors, and these positive behaviors are reinforced by frequent praise from all members of the community, both residents and staff members. Urine screens are random and frequent and even minor infractions are publicly exposed and punished. The explicit function of the social structure is to break down denial, pathology, and the code of the street, and to replace it with a code of responsibility, honor, trust, and helpfulness to each other. In this sense, the T.C. attempts to reparent residents by providing a good family—fair but demanding. Consistency in limit setting is a crucial ingredient.

While T.C.'s have always been physically nonviolent, the early T.C.'s were associated with verbal violence and the use of shaming and humiliating techniques (for example, sitting a resident to be punished in a corner with a dunce cap after his head has been shaved). Such harsh techniques were abandoned some years ago by virtually all T.C.'s and have been replaced by more positive and less physical methods of training the individual into being an honest contributing member of the community. However, in most T.C.'s, there are still encounters and marathon day-long meetings, during which verbal confrontation does take place. The individual is subject to stress and demand in the community, within the context of support and love.

Harbor House

Harbor House is a forty-five-bed T.C. located in the Bronx, New York. It was created expressly for homeless drug abusers who also have a major mental illness. The sponsoring agency, Argus Community, Inc., is a highly regarded drug treatment agency that has been actively working with a variety of populations in the South Bronx for twenty-five years. In 1985, responding to the growing number of homeless persons in New York City, Argus opened a T.C. for substance abusers who were also homeless. This program, Argus IV, has been successful in rehabilitating homeless addicts and currently serves forty-five men in its two-year-long residential program. However, like traditional T.C.'s, it does not accept addicts who are also mentally ill.

In 1987, the director and senior staff of Argus decided to create a new program for mentally ill homeless substance abusers. They contacted The Information Exchange (TIE), a training and consultation organization that has focused on working with clinical agencies in both the mental health and substance abuse fields to increase sharing of knowledge between them. Senior Argus clinical and administrative staff, working with TIE consultants, spent a year planning Harbor House, a modified T.C. specifically for seriously mentally ill addicts. The modifications, put as simply as possible, consisted of softening the hard edges of confrontation of the T.C., and integrating a mental health treatment team with the drug abuse counselors.

In a certain sense developing the clinical program was not the hardest part. It took over a year to get the three separate New York State Departments of Mental Health, Alcoholism, and Substance Abuse to cooperate on licensing and financing. Persistence was as important as creativity in launching this dual program for a new patient population. The basic state residential license was obtained from the drug abuse agency, while a license for mental health treatment was obtained from the mental health agency. Funding was secured for different program activities from different state, federal, and municipal sources.

Harbor House opened in December 1988 with room for thirty-five men who were homeless, mentally ill, and substance abusers. It has since increased its capacity to forty-five men. The counseling staff consists of men and women who are themselves recovering from substance abuse. The program director and other key administrative staff are also recovering from addiction. The mental health team consists of a part-time psychiatrist, part-time psychologist, and full-time nurse and social worker. They are not in recovery from addiction. In addition, consultants have continued to train all members of the staff about the needs and clinical characteristics of dually disordered persons.

Physical Plant. The program is located in a small apartment house, built in the early twentieth century, in a South Bronx neighborhood noted for its high crime rate. The building itself was in very poor repair when the program opened, but it has been rehabilitated by the residents themselves.

Integrated Treatment Model. As the description earlier in this chapter suggests, the Harbor House program can be seen as a model of integrated treatment for substance abuse and mental disorder. Specialist staff with backgrounds in treating each of these categories of disorder are cross-trained to at least understand treatment provided by other members of the integrated team. Many efforts are made to minimize the potential for conflict between the T.C. substance abuse treatment model and the model of psychiatric treatment by an interdisciplinary mental health team. Compromises have been developed by consensus when they are deemed necessary. For example, a particular patient may receive individual mental health counseling to support him in being able to tolerate and benefit from substance abuse treatment; or a person undergoing a period of severe psychiatric disturbance may be allowed more time in bed "resting" than would ordinarily be allowed for the resident of a T.C.

The program psychiatrist and psychologist conduct initial and periodic reassessments, review the diagnoses from prior hospitalizations, and manage medications. The majority of residents are maintained on psychopharmacologic medications, a distinct departure from the typical substance abuse T.C., where medication is not allowed. Senior psychiatric consultation is available when desired. Attempts are made to reduce or eliminate medications, but the majority remain on lowered doses.

Laboratory testing and emergency hospitalization are available through affiliation agreements between Harbor House and local psychiatric programs. When a patient becomes psychotic, which is an occasional but not common event, the patient is almost always able to return to Harbor House after a brief hospitalization.

The mental health staff, besides prescribing and monitoring psychiatric medications, also provide individual therapy on an as-needed basis. In addition, the mental health staff sit in on group counseling sessions conducted by the substance abuse counselors. Case conferences on interesting or difficult patients are conducted periodically for the entire combined staff by an outside training consultant who is a senior psychiatrist experienced in dual diagnosis treatment.

With regard to addiction treatment, Harbor House attempts to integrate the standard T.C. treatment approach with the less harsh and more accepting approach of the Twelve-Step self-help recovery programs such as AA and NA. Twelve-Step meetings are held at Harbor House a few times a week and groups of residents are also assisted and encouraged to go to outside community meetings at other times.

Mandated Abstinence. Harbor House is an unlocked and voluntary program, but is locked to the street, so that street addicts who are not in recovery cannot easily enter to steal the furniture and television sets. There is a firm expectation that the resident will remain drug and alcohol free during his entire stay. A condition of remaining in the program is that a resident must submit to a urine test if there is any suspicion that he may have used an illicit substance. Refusal to take such a test is tantamount to admitting that such a substance has been used. A positive test or a refusal to provide a urine sample for testing is grounds for immediate discharge.

A resident who has been discharged for drug use or who has left in order to use drugs may apply for readmission, but return to this community is not easy or automatic. This difficulty of return makes residents think long and hard before they give up their place at Harbor House by relapsing to drug use.

Admission Policy. Prospective residents are recruited from either New York City shelters for the homeless or from psychiatric hospitals that are seeking to discharge a male patient with a history of major mental illness and substance abuse, who is felt to require a structured residence such as Harbor House. Because of the funding requirements of the state, all prospective residents must have had documented homelessness and lived in a New York City shelter prior to their hospitalization. The only exclusion criterion is current, overt psychosis. Past history of criminal behavior is no contraindication to acceptance. Many of the residents have served time in municipal and state prison and a few have been convicted of homicide.

Who are the residents of Harbor House? An external evaluation was performed to provide information for a course at the annual meeting of the American Psychiatric Association in May 1990. At that point there had been 102 persons admitted to Harbor House; 67 had left for a variety of reasons, while 35 had stayed. All of those admitted met the three criteria of: (1) experiencing a polysubstance abuse or dependence; (2) being homeless at the time of admission or, if admitted directly from a psychiatric hospital, having been homeless prior to that hospitalization; and (3) having had at least two psychiatric hospitalizations and a diagnosis of a major mental disorder.

The majority of residents are African-American; there is a substantial minority of persons of Hispanic background and a small minority of persons of Caucasian background. The counseling staff are largely Afro-American and Hispanic, while several of the mental health professionals and consultants are Caucasian. The issue of race and ethnicity does not appear to present a problem in the operation of the program; the overriding similarity of concerns and interests appears to minimize the significance of ethnic differences.

Discharge Policies. One reason for discharge by the program is severe and active exacerbation of psychosis that requires hospitalization. A minor psychotic episode that is not accompanied by suicidal or homicidal risk is usually treated by the program. The only other reason for discharge is a substance abuse relapse.

Positive discharge is a planned event that typically occurs after eighteen to twenty months in the program. A careful and complete aftercare program is planned, including continuing connection to the Harbor House community. Employment, housing, and medical and psychiatric care are all arranged in advance.

Behavioral infractions are dealt with by program restrictions within the T.C. structure (see case example).

Motivation. The primary reason that individuals accept admission to Harbor House and stay—despite the stringent demands of the program and the unavailability of substance abuse as a coping mechanism—is that they view Harbor House as necessary for their survival. One resident of Harbor House describes having accepted admission "because I had hit bottom and there was nothing else for me to do but come to Harbor House or die." Prior to coming into the program, a typical resident oscillates between the street, shelters for the homeless, jail, and mental hospitals. Many of their peers in those environments die of drug addiction or of

AIDS. Because of the widespread prevalence of drug use and abuse in the shelter population, it is clear to the shelter resident that being sober and straight requires leaving that environment. Even the hospital is not necessarily drug free; many residents report that they were able to continue to drink alcohol or use illicit drugs while in hospitals, as well as while in prison.

Case Example. Robert was admitted to Harbor House early in 1989, voluntarily, from a shelter for the homeless. At the time of admission, he was a twenty-six-year-old single African-American male who had had four psychiatric hospitalizations. He had been discharged with the following diagnoses: (1) paranoid schizophrenia (Axis I), (2) polysubstance abuse or dependence (Axis I), and (3) antisocial personality disorder (Axis II). Principal substances used were crack/cocaine, marijuana, and alcohol. He was briefly in a drug rehabilitation program in 1985, at age seventeen. Earlier history of drug abuse treatment is not known. He was on five years probation, and had served time at Rikers Island, a New York City Corrections Department facility.

Psychosocial history: Mother was a drug addict. Little is known of his early childhood. He was raised in a foster family with several other children. At age nine he was a member of a group of children who were found to be engaged in seriously inappropriate sexual behavior. He has been convicted of rape and also reports that he was the victim of a homosexual rape while in prison. He reported that he has never been able to talk to women because of his shyness. He has made money as a male prostitute in order to buy drugs.

Adjustment in the residence: Robert had a hard time adapting to life in the T.C. but did not give up. His problems included poor concentration, confusion, occasional paranoid thinking, and significant difficulties with memory. He also showed attention-seeking behavior, poor communication skills, and deficient social and vocational skills. He was somewhat isolated from the other residents, and sometimes reported feeling that he was being picked on. At times, he believed that he had certain "powers"—for example, that when someone changed chairs in the room it was because his thoughts caused that person to move. While in the residence he stole food and cigarettes in such a way that he obviously would get caught. These behaviors were very childlike. When caught with stolen food in his hand, he has persisted in denying the theft.

Progress: After Robert had been a resident for ten months, he was placed back at the Orientation level (admission level) because of various infractions of house rules. After several weeks, he was subjected to a "probe" to determine his readiness to move on to the next level. Although he failed the "probe" and was therefore kept at the Orientation level, his response to this incident was positive: He immediately requested another probe, believing that he would be able to do better and thus advance to Level 1. This was a positive sign of his improved self-esteem and increased ability to relate to the rules and procedures of the residence.

The staff noted other positive changes during this time period. For instance, he began enthusiastically participating in the twelve-step self-help program of NA. His relationships with staff and other residents were also improving, and he sought reassurance and approval in a more socially appropriate way. For example, he asked a staff member whether he was going to get kicked out of the residence and was pleased with the assurance that he would not be asked to leave if he kept trying to improve. Moreover, he has accumulated several thousand dollars in his bank account from disability payments, and responded to this knowledge with a decision to stay in the residence. He stated that he was aware that if he were to leave the program prematurely he would use the money to buy drugs and get into trouble again.

Discussion: In reviewing this case for both psychopathology and personality immaturity, the staff made the following observations: (1) Personality growth has taken place since Robert entered the program. He can now be better contacted on an interpersonal level. He seeks attention and praise, and people feel good when they help him because of his response. Although he expresses doubts about his potential, he also expresses a wish to learn, grow, and become more capable. (2) Staff described Robert as being very immature and childlike at the time of admission. Specifically, he was seen as having: low frustration tolerance; extreme difficulty working persistently for a deferred goal (though some improvement had been noted in recent weeks: he was able to work at tiling a bathroom for more than an hour without giving up); shallow affect; tendency to lie to avoid punishment; extreme rejection sensitivity; tendency to test limits frequently. (3) His Global Assessment score had improved from 33 at admission to 65 one year later. Staff consensus was that although this young man of twenty-seven is developmentally immature, and in many ways functions like a five-year-old, growth and development appear to be under way. It was felt that he probably would not be ready for totally independent living—even after eighteen months to two years in the residence—but he would be a good candidate for a supportive apartment program after graduation.

Outcome Research

In September 1990, Argus Community Inc., was awarded a five-year research grant from the National Institute on Drug Abuse. An external research group will compare Harbor House outcomes against outcomes for the same population treated in traditional community residences operated within the mental health system. This carefully controlled study should provide valuable information about what works and what does not work in the treatment of such dually disordered individuals. Even before the research is completed, however, we can offer the following clinical observations, based on the first two years of Harbor House operation, to provide guidance for those who wish to develop similar programs:

Mentally ill substance abusers in a T.C. setting have psychotic relapses, but far fewer than would be expected if they were still using street drugs. Many are mild and can be handled within the program by medication adjustment, reduced demands, and increased support.

When relapses that require rehospitalization have occurred, most patients have been able to return to Harbor House after a brief inpatient stay in a cooperating community hospital.

Residents frequently express extreme gratitude for the integrated treatment approach. Many note that they were aware, in their prior experiences in psychiatric settings or substance abuse settings, that they were only being partially treated.

While in the T.C., most residents exhibit substantial personality growth and development, and consequent reduction of personality pathology.

Programs such as Harbor House are expensive, costing $35,000 per resident per year. Only one out of three patients admitted completes the program. However, while the program is more costly than a standard T.C. or residence for the mentally ill, its cost is still less than half that of state hospital care.

The psychiatrist and psychologist who have come to the program have been readily accepted by the counseling staff, even though they have not had the prior experience of recovering from substance abuse or of working in drug treatment agencies. The mental health professionals have found the work exciting, enjoyable, and professionally satisfying. They have developed great respect for the skills and dedication of counselors.

While the street outside is dangerous, because this part of the Bronx is a high crime and drug use area, once one enters Harbor House there is an attitude of safety, fun, and calm. The house is a comfortable and pleasant place in which to live, work, or visit.

In general, this treatment model appears to be effective as an integrated structural response to the "dual" needs of the clients.

Because Harbor House is such an expensive program, it clearly cannot be made available to all dually diagnosed individuals. It is hoped that ongoing research will further clarify which clients require—and can most benefit from—this expensive and intensive kind of treatment, and may offer guidelines for better patient selection in order to reduce the high dropout rate. Harbor House is not the solution for all dually diagnosed clients. Nonetheless, it does appear to merit further investigation and replication as a treatment approach of last resort for the most seriously troubled dually diagnosed individuals.

Reference

Campbell, R. *Psychiatric Dictionary.* New York: Oxford University Press, 1989.

Peggy McLaughlin, M.S.W., J.D., is a professor of social work at Ramapo College in Mahwah, N.J., and teaches around the country on issues of women and mental health.

Bert Pepper, M.D., has concentrated on learning about psychiatrically ill young people for the past twelve years. Much of his work has focused on developing new systems of care for the dually diagnosed.

The special problems of the dually diagnosed homeless are addressed in a mental health case management agency through two complementary treatment models, each with specific advantages.

Contrasting Integrated and Linkage Models of Treatment for Homeless, Dually Diagnosed Adults

John Kline, Maxine Harris, Richard R. Bebout, Robert E. Drake

The prevalence of substance disorders has risen dramatically among the population of severely and persistently mentally ill adults in the last ten years (Drake and Wallach, 1989). Accompanying this trend is an increase in housing instability and homelessness among this same group (Bachrach, 1984). Approximately 10 to 20 percent of the homeless are dually diagnosed, with concurrent major psychiatric and substance disorders (Tessler and Dennis, 1989). As treatment complications posed by the co-occurrence of major psychiatric and substance disorders have become evident, models for providing concurrent and integrated treatment for the dually diagnosed have been developed (Minkoff, 1989; Osher and Kofoed, 1989). Similarly, intervention strategies for the homeless mentally ill have been implemented with demonstrable success (Burwell and others, 1989; Harris and Bachrach, 1990). However, the effectiveness of a specific model of treatment for homeless, dually diagnosed adults has yet to be demonstrated.

Currently, clinicians working in the mental health system with dually diagnosed clients must choose between two treatment models: the *integrated model*, providing substance abuse treatment and psychiatric treatment within one integrated hybrid program, and the *linkage model*, linking patients in an integrated way to outside substance abuse programs. At Community Connections, a private, nonprofit case management agency in Washington, D.C., both these models are being adapted for work with homeless, dually diagnosed adults. The two models share a number of characteristics: Both rely on intensive case management, a continuum of residential services, and extensive psychosocial rehabilitation and socialization programs (Teague, Schwab, and Drake, 1990). In addition, both utilize a developmental perspective on dual diagnosis treatment that describes four phases in the progress of substance abuse treatment for dual diagnosis patients—engagement, persuasion, active treatment, and relapse prevention (Osher and Kofoed, 1989)—and both define treatment interventions that are phase-specific in nature. However, the two models are quite distinct in their approach to providing actual substance abuse treatment to dual diagnosis clients in each phase.

Integrated Treatment Model

The integrated treatment model provides for the treatment of both disorders simultaneously by consolidating mental health and substance abuse treatment under one supervisory and administrative umbrella. The integration of mental health and substance abuse treatment is based on three premises. First, because the network of substance abuse services available in the community at large is designed to treat higher-functioning adults, it tends to be unresponsive to the needs of dually diagnosed clients. Second, when treatment is separated into two distinct systems of care, both case managers and clients face more difficulty in negotiating and coordinating services. Third, substance abuse treatment becomes more effective and accessible for dually diagnosed clients when it is delivered by clinicians trained in the mental health needs of the dually diagnosed.

The core of an integrated treatment program consists of groups designed to address the needs of dual diagnosis clients during each specific phase of treatment. Included in the treatment spectrum are engagement or psychoeducation groups, pretreatment or "active user" groups, active treatment or "abstinence-orientation" groups, and relapse prevention groups. Group work in integrated treatment provides peer interaction, feedback, and emotional support to promote the necessary social network changes and life-style modifications required to maintain abstinence.

Clinicians in integrated treatment have two functions: case management and direct service. Case management includes the development of consistent, continuous, and responsive care, active relationship building, aggressive outreach, and provision of concrete services. Direct service includes provision of substance abuse treatment through ongoing individual counseling and coleadership of substance abuse groups. Case managers colead groups consisting of clients in their own caseloads to facilitate the bonding that must occur for successful work to proceed.

Engagement. Engagement represents the initial stage of contact between client and case manager. Emphasis during engagement is on the provision of basic services (housing, medical care, income support), general help and companionship, crisis intervention, and perhaps detoxification. The engagement phase of treatment with homeless dually diag-nosed clients requires more aggressive outreach and takes longer than with less disaffiliated groups. Distrust of service providers and treatment ambivalence are powerful negative forces operating in the initial stages of contact between client and case manager. During engagement, attention is given to the development of rapport and trust that can overcome barri-ers to collaboration.

During engagement with homeless dually diagnosed adults, individual counseling is strongly emphasized and is the focus of considerable atten-tion and supervision. Individual counseling in this phase, however, may ignore the issue of substance abuse treatment. Since future successful work depends on the development of rapport and trust, clinicians must be careful not to prematurely introduce substance abuse treatment issues that might encourage defensive reactions. During the engagement phase, the integrated treatment case manager assesses the client's tolerance for more intensive, confrontational substance abuse treatment, then determines the type and intensity of tactics to be employed during the persuasion phase.

Persuasion. Persuasion denotes the process of helping homeless dually diagnosed clients to recognize substance abuse as a problem in their lives and develop a commitment to pursue more intensive forms of treatment. Individual counseling, psychoeducation groups, and pretreatment or "active user" groups are utilized in the persuasion process. Individual counseling encourages the client to develop insight into the relationship between substance abuse and other problems of living (residential instability, hospi-talizations, social isolation). Individual work also focuses on the identifi-cation of potential "leverage," such as better agency housing and more spending money, that might be used to induce clients to accept treatment.

Psychoeducation groups distribute information about the problematic nature of substance abuse. These groups focus on the negative physiologi-cal, emotional, and cognitive consequences of continued substance abuse. Because of their educational focus, these groups are particularly safe and nonthreatening for homeless dually diagnosed clients and can be utilized during periods when other more intensive approaches may be intolerable. The group culture emphasizes acceptance and encourages participants to process material in their own way.

Pretreatment or "active user" groups are the third component of per-suasion. These groups include clients whose substance use remains active and whose defenses (for example, denial, rationalization, and intellectu-alization) remain strong. Because mentally ill individuals are usually un-responsive to a confrontational approach, group leaders must balance identification of resistances and defenses with supportive encouragement and sensitivity to clients' individual vulnerabilities. Group support enables group members to acknowledge for themselves the negative effects of sub-stance abuse in their lives. Information on the damaging physical, emo-

tional, and cognitive consequences of substance abuse is frequently introduced. This focus on the negative attributes of substance abuse makes
available for group members an alternative explanation for the problems of
living they have experienced. Once the client can genuinely acknowledge
that substance abuse is a problem and that reduced use or abstinence is a
worthy goal to pursue, the clinical team can refer the client from persuasion
to active treatment.

Active Treatment. The focus in the active treatment phase is on attaining group support for abstinence, changing one's support network from a
substance abusing to non-substance abusing one, and developing social
skills and life-style modifications that enhance the capacity to remain
abstinent. Though psychoeducation group interventions continue to be
utilized to support the newly found commitment to treatment, the primary
interventions in active treatment are individual counseling and "abstinence-
orientation" groups. During this stage of treatment, clients' distress and
discomfort about their substance use motivates them to make a commitment to change. Consequently, they are more able to constructively utilize
available peer group support for abstinence.

Individual counseling and case management focuses on the development of coping skills that empower clients to control the behavioral, cognitive, and affective factors that have contributed to their substance abuse in
the past. Individual work also provides emotional support for the difficulties
of attaining abstinence. Case managers continue to carefully monitor the
appropriateness of residential placements, the decision to enter active
treatment perhaps necessitating a shift in residence to remove a client
geographically from a substance abusing social network or to reward the
client's new commitment to treatment with more desirable housing. A medication regimen of disulfiram may also be introduced.

Abstinence-orientation groups teach, practice, and reinforce the development of coping skills. These groups have members who are struggling
toward abstinence as well as members who are already abstinent. Because
all abstinence group members share a commitment to abstinence as a goal,
discussions of abstinence can be allowed to evolve with less direction and
more participation than in persuasion groups. Group support for abstinence plays a critical role in the long-term outcome of active treatment,
since a major objective of the group is the evolution of an abstinence
support network outside the agency.

Relapse Prevention. Relapse prevention has been identified as the
critical phase in successful substance abuse treatment (Marlatt and Gordon,
1985). While clients tend to progress at individual rates, this last phase of
treatment generally begins after six months of abstinence. At this time,
enthusiasm about abstinence often begins to wane, as clients fail to realize
the idealized benefits of sobriety. Individual work now focuses on developing alternative coping skills designed to master pessimism and discourage-

ment. Case management work emphasizes continued psychiatric stability, maintenance of a non-substance abusing social network, vocational placement, and drug-free residential housing.

Relapse prevention groups provide emotional support to maintain clients' commitment to abstinence during a time of negative affective shifts. These groups also reinforce coping skills designed to enhance the prospects for continued abstinence and encourage the maintenance of healthy network contacts among group members. As in the previous two phases of treatment, group support is the critical intervention. Without the feedback, emotional support, and network modifications that occur through group work, progress through treatment phases would not be accompanied by the necessary life-style and attitudinal changes that ensure continued abstinence.

Linkage Treatment Model

The linkage treatment model represents a straightforward application of clinical case management principles to the special needs of the homeless dually diagnosed. In this model, case managers assertively link clients to existing substance abuse services in the community. Clients receive the full array of clinical services, with the sole exception that no specialized substance abuse treatment is offered in-house. Instead, case managers devote their attention to identifying, referring, and monitoring substance abuse services provided by traditional community-based treatment programs that rely heavily on self-help approaches such as AA and NA. AA and NA promote abstinence of addiction as a disease process and emphasize abstinence, social support, and a sober environment as critical to the recovery process (Emerick, 1987).

Historically, the liability of the linkage treatment model has been the failure to establish adequate links between the two treatment systems. Barriers to effective collaboration exist at several levels (Drake, Osher, and Wallace, in press). At the systems level, mental health and substance abuse services are commonly administered by separate governmental agencies that are often in competition for the same dollars and are eager to protect their limited resources. At a minimum, this system schism creates additional steps for dually diagnosed clients who need to access both sets of services (Bachrach, 1987). At worst, clients encounter exclusionary admission policies that, in effect, deny the co-occurrence of substance abuse and serious psychiatric disorders (Ridgely, Goldman, and Willenbring, 1990). Furthermore, front-line mental health treatment providers are generally unsophisticated and largely untrained about substance disorders, and vice versa.

In the linkage model, case managers are selected for their commitment to the social recovery ideology. They work proactively to expedite referrals through advocacy and careful client tracking, and to establish and maintain collaborative relationships with substance abuse providers and programs. Case management efforts will also include the education of front-line substance abuse providers about severe psychiatric conditions and the importance of maintenance psychotropic medication.

The linkage treatment model assumes the existence of adequate and accessible substance abuse programming in the community. When such services are available, linkage treatment offers several potential advantages for certain segments of the dually diagnosed population, including those individuals who have experienced significant bouts of homelessness. First, substance abuse services, including AA and NA groups, are increasingly available to homeless persons through drop-in programs, emergency shelters, and soup kitchens. Linkage treatment case managers can work to preserve the AA connections that already exist rather than needing to develop new therapeutic/supportive relationships.

Second, resistance to traditional mental health treatment is frequently quite pronounced among persons who are homeless and mentally ill (Blankertz and Cnaan, in press), particularly with respect to accepting the patient role (Harris and Bachrach, 1988). Substance abuse services within a clinic for the seriously and persistently mentally ill may invite resistance and cause the homeless dually diagnosed to flee treatment. In contrast, the intensive case management model utilized in the linkage approach features community outreach and the provision of services in the field rather than in an office or clinic setting. Linkage to substance abuse services that emphasize self-help approaches over traditional, medically oriented treatment may be less stigmatizing and better tolerated. For many dually diagnosed clients, participating in AA is more acceptable and less stigmatizing than participating in mental health treatment. Additionally, twelve-step programs allow for a certain degree of anonymity and less interpersonal intensity, particularly in large "open" meetings where members can simply listen without being pressured to speak.

Third, homeless mentally ill persons are frequently contact-avoidant and easily overwhelmed by intense interpersonal stimulation. Case management expressly uses the clinical relationship primarily as a vehicle for motivating clients to accept recommended services and for accomplishing essential clinical tasks—not for direct clinical treatment. The added intimacy and emotional intensity demanded by the integrated treatment model for substance disorders may in fact lead to a number of negative outcomes for the dually diagnosed homeless population. These outcomes include flight from treatment by individuals with schizoid and/or paranoid adaptations, and regressive reactions among persons with pathological dependency features or borderline personality dynamics (Harris, 1990; Bebout and Harris, 1990). The use of outside substance abuse providers within the linkage treatment model may serve to diffuse some of the interpersonal intensity inherent in intensive case management and mitigate such undesirable outcomes.

Case management strategies vary as a function of multiple factors, such as degree of impairment, type and extent of prior substance abuse treatment, legal status, level of motivation, and individual capacity to work with a case manager in the development and implementation of a treatment plan. In addition, clients require different interventions at different phases of the recovery process (Osher and Kofoed, 1989).

Engagement. The linkage model is similar to the integrated model during the engagement phase, with case managers in both approaches devoting considerable amounts of time to building relationships through consistent and frequent brief contacts. Efforts are focused on gathering assessment data and on enumerating and addressing immediate needs, such as medical care, income, and housing supports. The provision of tangible assistance promotes the development of a long-term, supportive relationship that can be stabilizing in itself and lay the foundation for all future clinical work.

Persuasion. During the persuasion phase, case managers offer resource information, evaluate the appropriateness of specific referrals, and begin to develop ways to induce clients to seek or accept treatment. Goals during this phase include increased client awareness of the disabling effects of substance abuse and receptiveness to treatment. Substance use is monitored through self-report and toxicology screenings. Treatment contracts place contingent demands on clients seeking resources such as desirable agency housing, increased independence with respect to living circumstances, or control over personal spending. Participation in programs offering substance use information in a psychoeducational format is encouraged.

Active Treatment. Admission to a detoxification or inpatient program may mark the beginning of active treatment, depending on the degree of impairment and frequency of use. Community-based programs utilized during this phase include AA/NA self-help programs along with other treatment programs that feature more direct confrontation and insistence on abstinence. Referrals and monitoring require case managers to develop collaborative, informal contacts within the substance abuse treatment community. Urinalysis continues to be used, and clients may be asked to maintain signature cards in order to track their attendance at AA and to document compliance with treatment plan requirements. While some clients in active treatment may continue to require structured, supervised residential placement to support their efforts to achieve abstinence, others may be able to move gradually toward more independent living.

Relapse Prevention. During the relapse prevention phase, case managers employing the parallel treatment approach continue to monitor attendance and use periodic drug screens, but frequency of contact and monitoring interventions may decrease slowly. Case managers no longer need to involve themselves in accompanying clients to treatment meetings as new network supports become firmly established. Incremental moves toward independence are encouraged, as tolerated, but flexibility with respect to case management contact and residential placement allows for movement back toward structure and supervision, because progress is so rarely linear. Primary attention is now given to maintaining drug-free housing and expanding one's range of activities (leisure, work, and so on) within a non–substance abusing network.

Residential Spectrum

In both models, a spectrum of residential services must be available to address homelessness. Successful residential programming for persons with dual diagnoses depends on the availability of a continuum of adequately supported residential opportunities (Pepper, 1985). With a few significant modifications, to be discussed later, this residential continuum can be adapted to substantially meet the housing needs of dually diagnosed homeless persons as they progress through the four phases of substance abuse treatment.

Any residential continuum for the mentally ill must incorporate a range of options that vary along several dimensions simultaneously: pressure for growth (versus maintenance), level of demand, degree of structure, and length of stay (transitional versus long-term). For the dually diagnosed there must be programs with varying levels of tolerance for substance use, ranging from unlimited use to limited use to total abstinence. Component programs may include a stratified apartment program as well as a series of supervised group homes with different lengths of stay: thirty-day crisis residences, intermediate-stay transitional houses, and long-stay group homes with significant levels of structure and support but minimal expectations regarding movement toward more independence.

Although the component programs are functionally differentiated, residential progress and transfers throughout the continuum may be monitored through a central residential review conference that emphasizes maximum integration as well as rapid and flexible response to the clients' changing needs. Client flow through the residential continuum is generally toward increasing independence and decreasing levels of supervision. However, allowances are made for movement back toward the more restrictive end of the continuum as needed. Gently assisting clients to move from unrealistic housing preferences toward greater acceptance of more supervised residential care is often a goal of the residential care providers.

Modifying Housing for the Dually Diagnosed

To serve seriously mentally ill adults with histories of homelessness and past or current substance disorders, the housing continuum must be adapted by taking into consideration three special issues.

Safety, Security Needs. Some housing advocates argue that treatment demands should be given second-order consideration when working with the chronically homeless and that safe, secure housing is a basic human right that should be given top priority (Hopper, 1989). While controversy surrounds the concept of "wet" housing, characterized by a permissive stance toward intoxication, more liberal rules for the homeless and dually diagnosed are advisable, as compared to residential treatment for substance abusers who are domiciled and not psychotic (Baumohl, 1989; Blankertz and White, 1990). The provision of adequate housing may advance the engagement process, promote compliance with essential clinical tasks (such as medication visits), and increase receptiveness to substance abuse treatment (Drake, Osher, and Wallach, in press). These notions represent a major shift in policy from traditional residential programming for substance abuse that commonly mandates treatment compliance and sobriety as prerequisites for housing. On the other hand, many clients need and can tolerate abstinence-oriented housing. For others, a residential program with some limit setting and confrontation of substance use may be a useful setting in which to facilitate further progress toward abstinence.

Inclusiveness. Admission and discharge criteria must be more inclusive, since abstinence may be an unrealistic standard for most dually diagnosed residents during the engagement and pretreatment stages. Discharge policies that are too restrictive often guarantee early failure and serve to perpetuate residential instability. Training and supervision become increasingly important in order to sensitize paraprofessional, on-line staff in the residential program to the slow, cyclic nature of the recovery process, both from addictions and from the trauma of homelessness.

Time Limits. Because the dually diagnosed homeless individual presents multiple deficits that slow the treatment process, the usual time limits imposed by transitional housing must be stretched. Residential moves, even positive ones toward increasingly attractive and independent housing, represent further stressors. Accordingly, transitions necessitated by administrative factors such as arbitrary time constraints, rather than by clinical needs, should be avoided. At the same time, homeless persons often exhibit a distinct pattern of rootlessness and restlessness, even when engaged in treatment (Harris and Bachrach, 1990), suggesting that transitional housing can play an important role. Further research is needed to illuminate the relative advantages and disadvantages of transitional versus permanent housing (Drake, Osher, and Wallach, in press).

Conclusion

Two prominent models of treatment for homelessness and dual diagnosis are commonly utilized by clinicians and program planners. The linkage treatment model provides a full range of clinical case management services to treat psychiatric disorders while pursuing a program of aggressive out-reach and referral to community substance abuse resources. The model emphasizes the significance of social networks in the maintenance of addic-tive behavior and employs aggressive interventions to change the nature of client social networks.

The integrated treatment model provides the full range of clinical case management services while also offering comprehensive substance abuse treatment in-house. This approach emphasizes intensive group work coor-dinated with individual counseling. The model assumes that an integrated approach compensates for the fragmentation between psychiatric and sub-stance abuse treatment systems in the community.

Both models have advantages and disadvantages. The integrated treat-ment model provides a unitary system of care that focuses on individual counseling and peer group cohesion; however, the interpersonal intensity of this model can be threatening and unacceptable to homeless dual diag-nosis clients. Furthermore, resistance to treatment and identification with the patient role is pronounced among the homeless, and the location of substance abuse treatment in a psychiatric setting is unappealing to many homeless clients.

The linkage treatment model emphasizes aggressive outreach to com-munity resources. This approach has a number of advantages. First, it recognizes the supportive relationships homeless people have developed through AA/NA groups already operating in the shelter system and the wisdom of keeping these linkages intact. Second, the emphasis on network linkages in the treatment of substance abuse allows homeless clients the opportunity to avoid the identification with the patient role mentioned previously. Third, the diminished degree of case management contact and interpersonal stimulation complements the contact-avoidant characteristics of many homeless clients and provides them a safe treatment environment. However, the linkage treatment model can ensure neither that substance abuse services are actually delivered nor that they are responsive to the clinical needs of the dually diagnosed.

The models are not mutually exclusive. They have applicability depend-ing on the individual characteristics of a referred client. The degree of willingness of clients to engage within an agency setting, bond with a case manager, and accept intensive treatment determines the appropriateness of referral to one or the other treatment approach.

These models may also be used sequentially. The less demanding, more diffuse substance abuse treatment approach of the linkage model can provide the only tolerable form of treatment for clients who are actively abusing substances and in a state of denial about their negative conse-quences. As the commitment to abstinence grows, the integrated approach can then be utilized to provide the intensive treatment and support clients may need to remain abstinent. As clients become more committed to abstinence and more engaged in AA, they may once again benefit from the linkage model in its emphasis on utilizing generic substance abuse treatment resources in the community.

References

Bachrach, L. L. "The Homeless Mentally Ill and Mental Health Services: An Analytic Review of the Literature." In H. R. Lamb (ed.), *The Homeless Mentally Ill.* Washington, D.C.: American Psychiatric Press, 1984.

Baumohl, J. Editor's Introduction to "Alcohol, Homelessness, and Public Policy." *Contemporary Drug Problems,* 1989, *16,* 281–300.

Bebout, R. R., and Harris, M. "Case Management Strategies for Long-Term Clients with Severe Personality Disorders." *TIE Lines,* 1990, *7,* 4–8.

Blankertz, L., and Cnaan, M. R. "Symbolic Interaction: A Framework for Outreach." *Social Casework,* in press.

Blankertz, L., and White, K. K. "Implementation of a Rehabilitation Program for Dually Diagnosed Homeless." *Alcoholism Treatment Quarterly,* 1990, *7,* 149–164.

Burwell, B. O., Dennis, M. L., Ethridge, R. M., Lubalin, J. S., Theisen, A., Fisher, P. J., and Schlenger, W. E. *Implementation Evaluation Design for NIMH McKinney Mental Health Services Demonstration Projects for Homeless Mentally Ill Adults.* Vol. 2: *Status Report of the Stuart B. McKinney Mental Health Services Demonstration Projects.* Research Triangle Park, N.C.: Research Triangle Institute, 1989.

Drake, R. E., Osher, F. C., and Wallach, M. A. "Homelessness and Dual Diagnosis." *American Psychologist,* in press.

Drake, R. E., and Wallach, M. A. "Substance Abuse Among the Chronic Mentally Ill." *Hospital and Community Psychiatry,* 1989, *40,* 1041–1045.

Emerick, C. D. "Alcoholics Anonymous: Affiliation Processes and Effectiveness as Treatment." *Alcoholism: Clinical and Experimental Research,* 1987, *2* (5), 416–423.

Harris, M. "Redesigning Case-Management Services for Work with Character-Disordered Young Adult Patients." In N. L. Cohen (ed.), *Psychiatry Takes to the Streets.* New York: Guilford Press, 1990.

Harris, M., and Bachrach, L. L. "A Treatment Planning Grid for Clinical Case Managers." In M. Harris and L. L. Bachrach (eds.), *Clinical Case Management.* New Directions for Mental Health Services, no. 40. San Francisco: Jossey-Bass, 1988.

Harris, M., and Bachrach, L. L. "Perspectives on Homeless Mentally Ill Women." *Hospital and Community Psychiatry,* 1990, *41,* 253–254.

Hopper, K. "Deviance and Dwelling Space: Notes on the Resettlement of Homeless Persons with Alcohol and Drug Problems." *Contemporary Drug Problems,* 1989, *16,* 391–414.

Marlatt, G. A., and Gordon, J. R. *Relapse Prevention: Maintenance Strategies in the Treatment of Addictive Behavior.* New York: Guilford Press, 1985.

Minkoff, K. "An Integrated Treatment Model for Dual Diagnosis of Psychosis and Addiction." *Hospital and Community Psychiatry,* 1989, *40,* 1031–1036.

Osher, F. C., and Kofoed, L. L. "Treatment of Patients with Psychiatric and Psychoactive Substance Abuse Disorders." *Hospital and Community Psychiatry,* 1989, *40,* 1025–1030.

Pepper, B. "Where (and How) Should Young Adult Chronic Patients Live? The Concept of a Residential Spectrum." *TIE Lines,* 1985, *2* (2), 1–6.

Ridgely, M. S., Goldman, H. H., and Willenbring, M. "Barriers to the Care of Persons with Dual Diagnoses: Organizational and Financing Issues." *Schizophrenia Bulletin,* 1990, *16,* 123–132.

Teague, G. B., Schwab, B., and Drake, R. E. *Evaluation of Services for Young Adults with Severe Mental Illness and Substance Abuse Disorders.* Arlington, Va.: National Association of State Mental Health Program Directors, 1990.

Tessler, R. C., and Dennis, D. L. *A Synthesis of NIMH-Funded Research Concerning Persons Who Are Homeless and Mentally Ill.* Rockville, Md.: NIMH Division of Education and Service System Liaison, 1989.

John Kline, M.S.W., is program director for substance abuse treatment at Community Connections in Washington, D.C.

Maxine Harris, Ph.D., is codirector of Community Connections.

Richard R. Bebout, Ph.D., is associate clinical director for residential services at Community Connections.

Robert E. Drake, M.D., Ph.D., is director of the New Hampshire–Dartmouth Psychiatric Research Center.

CONCLUSION

The preceding chapters have described an integrated conceptual framework for addressing the needs of dual diagnosis patients, and have outlined principles for designing comprehensive care systems, developing hybrid programs, and performing clinical assessments. Four innovative program models have been presented, each with uniquely creative, and potentially replicable, clinical interventions.

Despite the variation in the focus of each chapter and in the backgrounds of the authors, four common themes have emerged throughout the book:

1. *Integration.* Services provided for dual diagnosis patients, whether on a systems level, program level, or individual level, must develop a framework for integrating treatment of the psychiatric disorder with treatment of the substance disorder, both conceptually and clinically. Integration can occur both through the development of specific hybrid programs and through the linkage of more generic programs by systemic intensive case management.

2. *Comprehensiveness.* No one program model can serve the needs of all dual diagnosis patients, and even individual programs must have the ability to treat patients with a variety of clinical presentations. Dual diagnosis patients must be assessed to determine specific diagnoses and the phase of recovery and level of severity, disability, and motivation for treatment associated with each diagnosis. Specific program elements address patients at different phases: acute stabilization; engagement, education, and persuasion; active treatment to attain prolonged stabilization; relapse prevention and maintenance; and rehabilitation and recovery.

3. *Flexibility.* All systems and programs must be able to be as flexible as possible in modifying traditional treatment techniques—whether for addiction or mental illness—to address the unique needs of dual diagnosis patients. Such flexibility may range from providing detoxification services on a psychiatric unit or psychotropic medication in a detoxification unit, to developing a fully integrated cadre of dual diagnosis case managers, to incorporating a dual diagnosis group program into a traditional day treatment program.

4. *Continuity.* Successful treatment of patients with dual diagnoses requires continuity of treatment both longitudinally and cross-sectionally. Programs treating these patients must take into account their changing needs and symptoms, their propensity for lapses and relapses, and their long-term course. Patients commonly are treated in multiple programs in the course of recovery, and intensive case management is usually necessary to maintain a continuous focus among the various providers.

Hopefully these general guidelines will prove useful to clinicians, program managers, and system planners working to address the needs of dual diagnosis patients.

Kenneth Minkoff
Robert E. Drake
Editors

Kenneth Minkoff, M.D., is chief of psychiatric services at Choate Health Systems in Woburn, Mass., and medical director of the Caulfield Center, an integrated psychiatry and addiction hospital. He is on the clinical faculty of the Cambridge Hospital Department of Psychiatry of the Harvard Medical School.

Robert E. Drake, M.D., Ph.D., is associate professor of psychiatry at Dartmouth Medical School and director of the New Hampshire–Dartmouth Psychiatric Research Center.

INDEX

Ordering Information

New Directions for Mental Health Services is a series of paperback books that presents timely and readable volumes on subjects of concern to clinicians, administrators, and others involved in the care of the mentally disabled. Each volume is devoted to one topic and includes a broad range of authoritative articles written by noted specialists in the field. Books in the series are published quarterly in Fall, Winter, Spring, and Summer and are available for purchase by subscription as well as by single copy.

Subscriptions for 1991 cost $48.00 for individuals (a savings of 20 percent over single-copy prices) and $70.00 for institutions, agencies, and libraries. Please do not send institutional checks for personal subscriptions. Standing orders are accepted.

Single copies cost $15.95 when payment accompanies order. (California, New Jersey, New York, and Washington, D.C., residents please include appropriate sales tax.) Billed orders will be charged postage and handling.

Discounts for quantity orders are available. Please write to the address below for information.

All orders must include either the name of an individual or an official purchase order number. Please submit your order as follows:
  Subscriptions: specify series and year subscription is to begin
  Single copies: include individual title code (such as MHS1)

Mail all orders to:
  Jossey-Bass Inc., Publishers
  350 Sansome Street
  San Francisco, California 94104

For sales outside of the United States contact:
  Maxwell Macmillan International Publishing Group
  866 Third Avenue
  New York, New York 10022

OTHER TITLES AVAILABLE IN THE
NEW DIRECTIONS FOR MENTAL HEALTH SERVICES SERIES
H. Richard Lamb, Editor-in-Chief